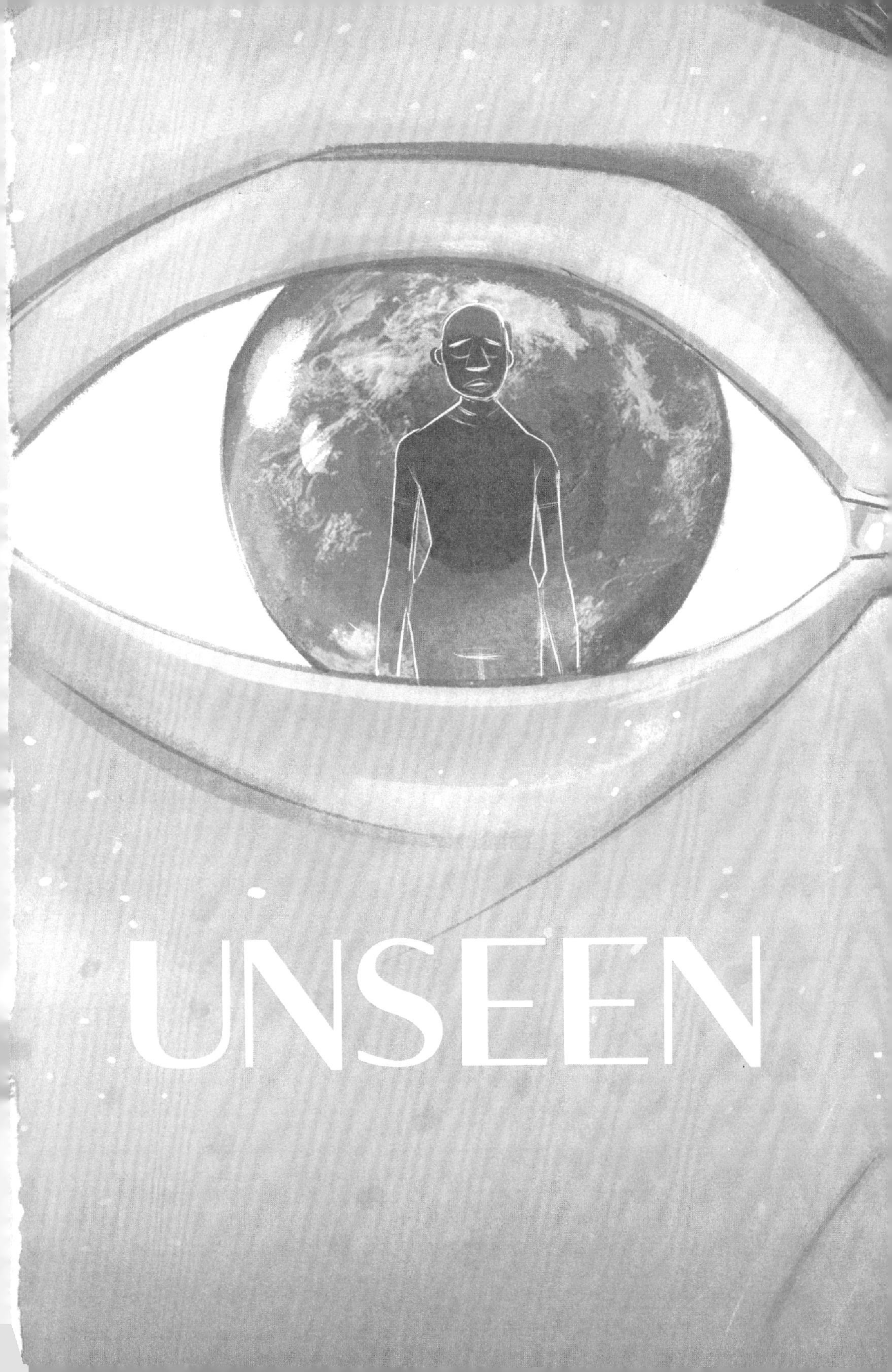
UNSEEN

UNSEEN

Field Notes of a Global Psychiatrist

Craig L. Katz

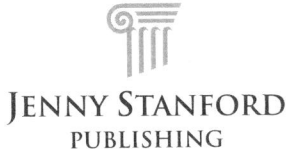

JENNY STANFORD
PUBLISHING

Published by

Jenny Stanford Publishing Pte. Ltd.
101 Thomson Road
#06-01, United Square
Singapore 307591

Email: editorial@jennystanford.com
Web: www.jennystanford.com

British Library Cataloguing-in-Publication Data
A catalogue record for this book is available from the British Library.

Unseen: Field Notes of a Global Psychiatrist

Cover Art: Created by Chase Walker

ISBN 978-981-5129-42-7 (Hardcover)
ISBN 978-1-003-56767-7 (eBook)

To
Linda, Maya, and Lev,
who give me the confidence to go places
and make me want to come back

Contents

Preface

The atmosphere is heavy here, but it's nothing physical. So much has happened that it's hard to get out from under history. So much needs to be done that it's hard to get out from under the present. And so much seems uncertain that the future barely has the traction to tug you in its direction.

The swirl of people on the dirt roads of the capital city rushes at me like so many currents at risk of sweeping me away in the undertow. This is no casual stroll. I am not even sure how I can be thinking of anything but my bearings, except that it is also a place that demands your attention, and I am nothing if not obedient.

Caution and curiosity team up, and I find myself wondering what it would be like to live one of the lives of the people around me, not my faraway life an ocean away back home. I came here on the leading edge of my life, but the immensity of this devastated country brushes me back. A lethal infectious outbreak, a civil war, and a typhoon—my comfortable life no longer feels like the default position but rather a privilege and a mirage.

I am walking in unwitting solidarity with a gentleman who is going my way, and I am tempted to throw my arm around his shoulders and make it official. But he walks slump-shouldered, and I imagine how it backfires and I drag both of us into the currents. He wears a baseball cap even though the sport has no place on this continent—a souvenir from family visiting from the U.S.? It shadows his face from the unrelenting sun, but I can see that the face has shadows of its own. He walks shoelessly on autopilot, lost in thought and unmoved by the movement around us. My comrade in arms wears a formerly white T-shirt lumbering its way toward the same tan color as his cap.

Everyone is said to have a twin, but I notice my walking companion's opposite coming our way. A man who I am tempted to call Dapper turns out of a doorway into the flow with the authority of a car steering into traffic. It's strange how formidable he seems despite being so trim. It's also said that clothes make the man, and his attire seems to be his secret—powder blue collared dress shirt and khaki pants are layered atop shoes whose blackness sparkle through the city's dust. A briefcase completes the ensemble. Dapper looks like he should be wearing thick, black-rimmed spectacles, but he seems sharp-eyed all on his own. It's the morning, and I imagine he is going to be right on time for work.

At this point my musings halt as a pick-up truck parts the sea of pedestrians, struggling to declare its supremacy over streets that should really outright belong to it and its automotive brethren. No one complains, gesticulates, or even seems to mind. Maybe when you have been bullied by the fates in the guise of warlords and typhoons you just go with the flow whenever you can and hope it goes with you.

People, all men, fill the truck's flatbed, standing together like toothpicks jammed in a jar. They are likely day laborers on their way to a rice farm. No one stumbles or falls out because no one seems able to move. There is no sense that anyone on the truck is holding onto their neighbor or looking out for them, but the sheer physics of the arrangement creates some interdependence. It is striking how people who not long ago fought one another in civil war can now stand on top of one another and think nothing of it. In fact, I wish I knew what they were thinking. Their impassive faces must be part of their work uniform and belie the livelier mental life that I hope lies within (and in fact intended to mask it).

The truck slows down and stubbornly stops right in the middle of it all when the driver notices a young woman whom I also notice because, like me, she is white. She bounds to the back of the truck and leaps onto the bumper, striking up a conversation with the passengers. After a minute she leaps back to the ground, unzips her knapsack, and tosses a few medicine bottles to them. Then she is back on the bumper as the men somehow find the leeway to pass the bottles between them under her watchful eye, ensuring that everyone gets one of what I would guess is antimalarial medication. The exercise ends with her running around and hopping into the passenger seat of the truck.

The woman is a relief worker—of that there is no doubt. The only questions are what malady brought her here and for how long. You could probably round out the essential facts of her relationship to it all if you also knew the aid agency she works for, summoned in the last six months following the typhoon. Up until then, the country had been embroiled in several years of civil war. Realists say it was a fight for control of the country's oil fields and that the religion each side cloaked itself in could be no religion if it sanctioned such biblical death and destruction.

The typhoon was in fact a blessing in disguise. It added to the carnage, but at least it was not man-on-man but an act of God that caught everyone's attention. The rains doused the fires raging in the bellies of the combatants. From my everyday vantage point right here on the street, I can look around at the one- or two-story storefronts and offices and almost instantly find the physical marks left by the natural disaster, especially a fuzzy brown line that the high-water mark of the floods crayoned across many of their facades. On the other hand, the woman relief worker surely symbolizes what else the rains left behind. Few relief agencies dared set foot in the country during the war, but most felt it safe enough now.

Most of the buildings on this street and indeed many streets in this city remained structurally intact despite the flooding. This long overdue good luck was, in the way of things here, offset by how badly the waters eviscerated the buildings and destroyed so much of their contents. The intact facades are at this point often just that— deceptively optimistic vestments.

Second-floor businesses were spared the direct impact of the floods so long as their first floors did not dissolve beneath them. On this morning, I look up and notice an herbalist's practice that seems to be in full swing. The country has for centuries turned to all manner of traditional healers, especially spiritual ones, to cure what ails the body and spirit of its people. Like umbrella salesman on a rainy day, faith healers in particular have seen a boom in their business since the typhoon seemed to bring if not God's wrath, then at least his rebuke; and if the intact buildings are to be believed, his mercy.

A child suddenly interrupts my navigation—through the streets and my thoughts—when she comes up to me to solicit my interest in buying fresh coconut water. Reluctant to eat or drink anything off the street here, I wave them off. I do try being as polite as one can be when saying no to a child because I know they are trying to help their families make ends meet or maybe even having to fend for themselves. The war left countless children orphaned and drove down the average age of the country. Adults killed one another off, and the elderly too often succumbed to the privations they faced.

I am new to the country and so can only guess what its children's lives are like right now. But the guesswork is easy. Theirs cannot be a child's life. Parents and caretakers are either absent or unable to provide for their families. Schools have only now begun to resume classes, even if with overflowing, underequipped classes. The war took their teachers' lives, and the typhoon their schoolbooks. And a sizable number of children who were conscripted as child soldiers have been asked to lay down their weapons and act like children again with a pittance of guidance on how exactly to do this. There just are not enough guides to help them demobilize nor enough knowledge anywhere in this world as to how exactly to beat swords into teddy bears.

Vendors of all kinds, selling fruit, clothes, and even chickens, line the sides of the street. There are no signs or fancy storefronts. I cannot even tell if anyone is ever in the same place twice or has a loyal clientele that would care. I bet there is a lot more going on around me than my foreign eyes can discern, let alone take in. I will say that the fruit sellers stand out to me, as they squat on tablecloths with fruit piled around them like sandbags around a foxhole. I sometimes imagine war breaking out again, and their resorting to hurling mangos like snowballs in defense of their turf. Such perverse humor, but I keep it to myself. The fruit vendors are also the exception to my prohibition against street food since I can buy bananas guaranteed fresh by Mother Nature with the peel that she has sheathed them in. I could peel the mangos, too, but they are just too messy.

I have long since left my walking companion in the dust, instead keeping pace with Dapper, who seemed to be going my way and with my Western pace. Stopping to buy some bananas eventually cuts me off from him, too, for the last leg of my walk. But when I finally arrive at the general hospital, they are both somehow there. It's like a finish line reunion. Dapper, looking like he could indeed run a marathon at any minute, is talking on his cell phone, perhaps one last personal call before diving into work. My other friend sits on the steps that usher visitors into the main entrance, lingering as though lost, afraid, or, I now wonder, unwell.

Acknowledgments

So many thanks go to Hara Estroff Marano without whose editing, ideas, and especially encouragement the idea for this book never would have gotten past the first three chapters. In that regard, thanks are also due to Grant Brenner, whose usual generosity and collegiality were on full display when he offered to look at those dust-gathered chapters and then introduced me to Hara so that I would write more. Along the way, Jacob Appel guided me on the ways of publishing and Vicki Gluhoski lent a cognitive behavioral psychotherapy lens to the book. Much gratitude also goes to the few and the proud who read original full-length versions of the book— Edith Karpf, Jerald Underdahl, Robert Frocarro, and Allison Bloom.

This book is about global mental health and would neither exist nor mean anything without the mental health work I have been privileged to engage in through the Mount Sinai Program in Global Mental Health. This privilege derives from the humility, hospitality, and foresight of our many liaisons around the world, particularly in Haiti, Saint Vincent and the Grenadines, Grenada, Belize, Guyana, the Dominican Republic, Liberia, Kenya, India, Nepal, Japan, and the United States. Experiences from these countries form the weave and the purpose of this book. Many visionary donors, big and small, have enabled us to string together our program and have these experiences over the years. And, from my very first day on faculty in 2000, so many leaders at the Icahn School of Medicine at Mount Sinai have given me the freedom, resources, and support to participate in disaster and global mental health. I have also been fortunate to be joined in this journey by so many wonderful students, residents, fellows, faculty, and program coordinators (Clement Kairouz, Megan Sacco, Kira Schmidt, and Peradeba Raventhirarajah), mostly from Mount Sinai and occasionally from other medical schools. But no one at Mount Sinai deserves more of my gratitude than Dr. Jan Schuetz-Mueller, my former resident-turned-co-director of the Program in Global Mental Health. His partnership and his poise mean the world to me and, I am sure, to the world.

In the end, no one deserves more thanks than my family. Marrying into my wife, Linda Chokroverty's, Indian family in a very real sense provided me with my first global experience following a sheltered suburban upbringing. And Linda has been a steadfast supporter of my global travel and aspirations ever since, including participating as a child psychiatrist herself. I have also been lucky enough to bring my children, Maya and Lev, on some overseas trips with me. I hope they know they are with me wherever I go.

Chapter 1

Sam

Sam felt bad. It was the peak of the sunlit afternoon, but for Sam it may as well have been bedtime. And it had been this way for weeks. He had begun to dread the inevitable drop off in energy that occurred like clockwork each day. Sam had also begun to fear his boss would find out. Jobs were scarce, and Sam used the energy of this fear to push himself day after day to farm and farm.

Rice farming has a comforting rhythm for those who know it. Clearing the land, seeding it, irrigating it, draining it, and harvesting it. The cycle takes four to six months. Sam's labor halts during the 2–3 months it takes for the seedlings to mature into harvest readiness. The irrigation period is about watching and waiting—mostly watching the perimeter to secure it from squatters while the farm experiences what is usually its quietist period. Provided enough time and water, Mother Nature does most of the work quietly and solemnly. For Sam, those 2–3 months are precarious ones when his income drops and he needs to find odd jobs or travel far from home to farms that are off-cycle from those in his town.

This was his hometown farm, and he had just returned to work the harvest after several months, waiting for the rice to grow. In the past, he worked the irrigation, but this time he decided the irrigation pay, or what one bookish friend called "irritation pay," was just too low. Suffering through a regular drop in pay may have been loyal to his boss, but it was disloyal to his family.

Unseen: Field Notes of a Global Psychiatrist
Craig L. Katz
Copyright © 2025 Jenny Stanford Publishing Pte. Ltd.
ISBN 978-981-5129-42-7 (Hardcover), 978-1-003-56767-7 (eBook)
www.jennystanford.com

Sam spent the last few months traveling back and forth to the capital city for work. The bus ride cost him time (three hours one way) and money ($USD 1.00/ride), but it was worth it. Sam operated a street-corner photocopy machine. And if he had a good day, he would make as much as $10/day before expenses. The tabletop machine belonged to the man who sold the rice seeds to the farm, who, on a recent trip to the U.S. to visit some cousins, inherited an old photocopier as a gift to bring back with him. He was not sure what a rice seed supplier could do with it, but he derived great pride returning home with such a trophy in hand.

Sam had been doing the seed deliveries for the supplier for the two weeks he was in America. The photocopier and a business idea insinuated themselves into their relationship when Sam took notice of the technology while returning the delivery truck keys after the trip. Sam agreed to operate it for him as a business, himself buying the supplies and doing the upkeep on the machine but in return, getting half of all the proceeds.

Sam had a friend who worked at a convenience store right in the heart of the capital, and the storeowner agreed to let Sam operate the photocopier on the bustling corner outside of the store, using the space and his electricity. For the former, he charged nothing, but for the latter, it would be $1 per day. It was a lot, but the photocopier might as well have been a rock and chisel without electricity. His friend got a free photocopy per day for his efforts.

Sam bought some paper and began street-side operations in earnest within a day. He perched the black machine on an upside-down cardboard box and ran a long electrical extension cord back into the store through an open window. Periodically the machine would just turn off, which proved not to be a mechanical error but rather the effect of someone's needing to plug in the blender to make a fruit shake for a customer.

One day the machine started producing faded copies, followed by blank copies. That is when Sam learned about ink toner and realized the machine was not as magical as he had wanted to believe. He found a store that could order the toner for a sum of $100, costing him nearly the entirety of his remaining profits. Even worse, it took a whole month to arrive. During that time, people began paying him 10 cents to put their face up against the glass, seeking to make a wish sure to come true in the bright flash of a toner-less turn of the machine. One supplicant got a seizure from the experience, but no one got their wish, leading demand to drop off within days.

After the arrival of the toner, the good times seemed to roll on, with Sam and his machine almost as popular as a street performer and his musical instrument. It all ended about a month later when a number of lights on the operations panel came on and the rest of the machine turned off. The blinking "Service Needed" crushed Sam's spirits, as there was surely no such technical expertise in his country, and even if there were, he could no longer afford to keep pouring money into his needy ward. He returned the machine to the rice supplier and himself to the farm as, fortuitously, harvest was at hand.

Working on the farm did not mean resting on it, and yet today Sam felt like lying down in the tall grains of the rice field. Whenever he looked from afar at the youthful green of a rice field in full growth, he had always imagined it was a feathery blanket. The image inevitably made him feel guilty about being paid to pluck the stalks and undo the weave. Today, the rice-field-as-blanket was more than idle fantasy, as he was tired in both mind and body.

In truth, Sam felt like hiding as much as he felt like sleeping. And even more, he felt like things were just happening to him. It was strange to him how magnetic the pull was to lie down right there, as though the earth's gravity was meant for him and only him. Even stranger, he did not care if he laid in the remaining inch of irrigation water that still stretched like a silvery top sheet over the expanse of ground as drainage proceeded.

When the typhoon swept in not a year ago, Sam and his countrymen acquired a weary respect for water. The volume and vigor of the torrents felt biblical, and Sam could not decide whether it was good or bad to be the subject of such divine attention. God had taken pity on them after years of endless civil war and sent the rains to drench the flames of war and just in case, the winds to blow them out.

But God was not letting them off easy, and the cure itself possessed its own poison. They mopped up the soaked country for so long it felt like the only purpose of drying it out was to generate new implements for further drying it out. The circularity of it all had made Sam wish the hand of God would again reach down and just wring out the whole country *en masse* into the nearby ocean. Water had been a friend turned enemy, and Sam shuddered at the sight of pooled water even after the cleanup more or less ended for him.

Now, Sam considered laying in the muck. This may have been spawned by another idea that had begun sneaking around in Sam's mind—that he deserved to be in the muck. It was hardly a central thought around which others orbited, but it was in play, nonetheless. Sam felt like a pig. Not being good enough for his wife and kids who now lived across the country with her parents had worn down his self-confidence, having whittled it down so much that it began to take his sense of self with it. Had you asked him outright, Sam could have honestly denied feeling like a pig and thought you absurd to ask. But don't doubt that the idea preyed upon him.

The predation was all the more troubling because it snaked around Sam's relationship with his scythe, the tool of the trade in rice harvesting. Sam questioned whether life was worth it. Whether his life was worth it. He had owned the same scythe for years, mostly out of financial necessity but also out of loyalty. At the harvest, it felt like an extension of his body. There was a time during the war that he even imagined himself as a superhero whose right arm ended in a scythe, empowering him to end the war in a truly single-handed fashion. It was a fantasy that bespoke the healthy self-confidence that farming, and especially harvesting, bestowed upon him. Now, he had wondered, albeit at a considerable distance from the thought, whether to turn the scythe on himself.

The good news was that Sam's scythe had begun to feel so heavy that slicing rice stalks now seemed like he was swinging one of the 50 lb bags of rice. Heavy, awkward, and impotent. Swinging at a rice stalk with an industrial-sized bag of rice could be the stuff of comedy or even farce but not in these weighty circumstances.

Today fatigue finally won out over the rest of Sam's motivations, including the fear of losing his job, as Sam decided he could not work another moment. But instead of slinking to the ground, Sam wandered off to the equipment shack as though to use the exposed toilet that occupied one of its corners. He never used it but instead went around back where wild grass indigenous to desolate places nuzzled the wall. Sam laid down in the angle of the wall. He was curled up on his side, back to the wall, the crushed grass his mattress and his ball cap the pillow.

It was a relief to give up his body to the earth, which handled the weight without fanfare. Sam remembered learning about gravity before he dropped out of school and wondered for a moment why we spend our every waking moment fighting it. The nihilism of this escaped him, as did the fact that he never used to think this way.

Maybe it was fear of being found out or the brightness of the equatorial sun, but Sam just could not sleep. It made no sense to him to have wasted the luxury of this break, making it feel doubly sinful. Neither work, nor rest. In fact, he paid for the indolence of his body with over-activity of the mind. It was not Sam's way to think about his "mind," but he was aware that his thoughts, bad thoughts about himself as a worker, a man, a father, and a husband would lay siege if given the chance. Quiet time had become the enemy and self-recrimination its henchmen.

Sam went back to work, having at least evaded the notice of his boss. Now the toil and monotony of rice farming came as a relief. Trying to regain mastery of his leaden body became a welcomed challenge, like riding a recalcitrant horse. He rode it all the way to the end of the day when he could finally get relief from having to deal with the afflictions of his body and mind.

Sam walked with his fellow laborers to their after-hours haunt, a street-side shack that served wine distilled from the sap of local palm trees and meat over boiled rice. Being able to eat the fruit of their labor counted for something. The men sat on milk crates and played cards in between swigs. Their evening usually began in tired silence and ended with rowdy debates about the national football league and political scandals.

Sam drank freely but forced himself to eat his dinner. His usual appetite for food had faded while his thirst for alcohol escalated. He ate his meal out of respect for God and to his hard-earned income. His friends began to notice.

"Hey Sam, what's da mata, bro? I done see you take rest today."

"I don't know, man, but tanks."

"You don't feel good—yo body?"

"No, brotha. It's not right by me right now."

"Man, you need to see Londo. Have you seen Londo?"

"No. I got it."

"Maaannn… you don't got it no how. You gotta see him."

Dinner cleared out sooner than usual that night, and Sam found himself sitting alone atop his milk crate. The other crates seemed to be awaiting some words of consolation from him in the face of their abandonment. An unseen hand had turned on the moonlight, and it cast shadows over the crates, revealing an elegance that hid in daylight. The tropical sun just faded their fluorescent colors and then cruelly highlighted the decay and the dust in which it was encrusted.

The moonlight was not so kind to Sam, who looked, and felt, lonely and decrepit. He sat hunched over, feet planted, elbows on knees, and cheeks in hands. You would have thought he had fallen improbably asleep for the night but for the life in his eyes. They scanned the scene and sparked in the light. His mind was not nearly so active, mostly idling at lonely. In fact, passivity made up his most active thought. He wished to be able to stay, go nowhere, do nothing.

Sam's mind eventually wandered to his dinner partner's advice about Londo. Londo was the healer most people in their village trusted. There were a few other healers, but no one really took them seriously. They were regarded as the people you saw if you could not afford Londo. Londo was himself a farmer by day and did his healing late into the night. Everyone seemed to be able to find Londo when they needed him, whether he was in the fields or at his undistinguished-looking home clinic. Sam figured he would wander over, getting up as though he had an Olympic barbell on his shoulders and lumbering his way there as though he never put it down.

Londo operated out of a single room whose walls were ringed by rickety brown bookcases devoted to books, plants, palm fronds, citrus fruits, threads, candles, and ointment bottles. There was a desk off to the side that itself housed a number of small plants that looked like they were probably also tools of the trade. After waiting on a plastic lawn chair just outside the door in the sticky dusk, Sam sat down opposite Londo. They sat on two floor pillows under light cast by a table lamp and an enormous candle.

Londo opened, "What gives wit you, my friend?"

Sam explained his friend told him to come. "I can't get no energy."

Londo told him to hold out of his hands and looked them over, palm up and then down. He wanted to know whether Sam was having problems with erections.

Sam indignantly but dishonestly waved that off. "Hey Londo, dat jus not my problem."

"You play footboll, yeh?"

"I do not. Can't no way. I am like a plant out there—guys just go around me. Last time I played, we lost 5-0, and it was because of me."

"Hey. Football is a team sport, friend. How could it all be your fault?... Were you that good before? No goals for your team because you can't score?? Hah!"

"I tell you, it's me. I am no good for nuttin. That's all I am good for—nuttin. Can't farm, can't play."

"Yo, didn't you just say the women were no problem? You good for something!"

"Yeah... I got dat," admitted Sam while admitting otherwise to himself.

A great idea snapped Londo to his feet. He grabbed a palm frond and stood over Sam. Holding it with two hands like a sword, Londo tapped Sam's and his head with its large leaf five times back and forth. Next came a flask of something unnamed for Sam to drink. Its bitter taste was encouraging.

Londo sat back down and asked hopefully, "How do ya feel?"

Sam gave it a thought and ignoring his doubts, offered, "I think you done me good, but maybe I need to wait to feel it."

Londo agreed, advising him to give it a few days.

"So, what I got?" Sam mustered. He was unsure if he would have to pay extra for the answer.

"You got too few vitamins. I give them back to you."

"How did I get that?"

"Too much work, too little church. You been goin' to church?"

"No."

"Your family still up-country, no? When they return?"

"Soon." He had no idea.

After a silence, Sam paid and plodded toward the door. His feet were fending for themselves while a question poked at him like a mosquito: "What's the point?" He tried shooing away the nonsense with a feeble shake of the head.

Sam dropped back into the plastic lawn chair that made up Londo's curbside waiting room with such abandon that it creaked in near collapse. As the darkness stared back apathetically, a young couple soon arrived hand-in-hand to see Londo. The man was mumbling to himself and stopped suddenly at the threshold to Londo's study, his momentum backing up into a brisk series of sideways and over-the-shoulder glances. His wife seemed half his size but with a weary declaration, "It okay, my Berko," forged inward and dragged him along. The man's frightened gaze led Sam to diagnose who really needed the healing, and self-doubt linked arms with the commotion to eject Sam into the night.

Chapter 2

The Missionary

The room is wall-to-wall white, but the air is red hot. I search for the remote control for the air conditioner that waits quietly for its marching orders. Anticipating its eviction, the heat seems to grab at my arms and legs to hold me back. It is no contest, and I drop into the bed as the air conditioner whispers its promise of relief. A poster looks back at me and declares, "We Da People," one word in red, one in green, and one in black.

Hotel rooms in the developing world somehow always have this same smell—smokey sweet. I have thought about this and am pretty sure it is the atmospheric effect of the endless fires for cooking across the landscape layering on top of the earnest cleaning efforts of the proprietor. I wish I could bottle the humility and bring it back home.

Just as familiar is a thought that somehow reaches around to punch me in the gut—"What am I doing here?" I await the work trip that does not begin with doubt, especially since planning for my travel should already have asked and answered the question, "Why am I going there?" I look at the photo of my wife and young kids on my phone and know I am not flattering myself when I read the question on their minds—"Why did you have to leave again?"

Unseen: Field Notes of a Global Psychiatrist
Craig L. Katz
Copyright © 2025 Jenny Stanford Publishing Pte. Ltd.
ISBN 978-981-5129-42-7 (Hardcover), 978-1-003-56767-7 (eBook)
www.jennystanford.com

I am a psychiatrist who works in global health. A chance opportunity to help out grieving families after a major airline crash killed all aboard many years ago inspired me to get more involved in this novel area of practice. I started organizing psychiatrists to help other disaster-affected communities but soon saw how responding to overseas disasters such as tsunamis and earthquakes was usually too little and too late for mental health needs since most countries around the world barely have any psychiatric services in the first place. This was brought home to me when an elementary school teacher in a tsunami-stricken town stood up and thanked us for our lecture on how to identify trauma-related mental health needs in their students and then asked where we were before. Most of the world is a disaster when it comes to mental health even without being stricken by one.

Mental health problems are the health problems that cause the most suffering, or what we call in medical-speak "morbidity" in the world, and yet most of them go unnoticed. And even when they get to the point of calling attention to themselves, the will and the means for dealing with them seem to reside on the head of a pin already cramped with those dancing angels. I have never met a minister of health or hospital executive who would say mental health care was unimportant but have never seen a health care budget that says mental health care is important. So, I shifted my focus away from global crisis response toward improving access to mental health care in day-to-day life and started a program in what we call global mental health. Most people think of AIDS or kids with diarrhea when they think of global health, but my program bucks the trend. Psychiatric colleagues that I have recruited for the cause and I fly around the globe to try to fill in what those in the know call "the mental health gap"—the chasm between the level of mental illness on this earth and the resources to address it. I do this because people and communities are more productive when you reduce the burden of their mental illness. And beyond what people do and how they contribute is how they feel—not all mental illness disrupts someone's functioning, but it always causes suffering. I want to do my part to reduce that suffering and make the world a happier place.

While most of us in our global mental health program treat individual patients back home, but when go abroad a community or country is our patient. To try to treat individual patients ourselves would be futile. Instead, we work by training, supervising, educating, advocating, and organizing—trying to leave behind better knowledge about, concern for, and comfort with mental health care across the strata from community members to health care providers to government officials.

We are mental health missionaries, but my host, Dr. Mary Juma, would be a mental health angel. She embodies the kind of point person we count on in a partner country to make our work possible. In fact, we count on them to draw our attention to their country in the first place—these things should be by invitation only and not borne of what some naysaying colleagues call "medical imperialism." Offering unbidden help to a country or community with their mental health needs often flops as readily as do my attempts to help someone dragged into my office by a spouse. Best to think of oneself or one's community as the patient and not be told you are one.

So, my arrival here was the culmination of a process that goes like this: first, a colleague from another partner country recommends my program to Mary the way a satisfied patient recommends me to a new patient; she emails me, and we have some electronic back and forth that hints at the promise of a partnership (global mental health could barely exist without the ease of communication permitted by email); we talk by audio or video and decide there is indeed a potential match between what my program has to offer and what her country needs; we revert to email to work out the logistics of a trip; and then here I am trying to gauge how to realize that potential. A drive to do good meets a need to do better.

Mary picked me up from the capital city airport earlier this afternoon, adding chauffeur to her overflowing portfolio—"Ahh... welcome good doctor, to our country. I trust you had a good flight?" She introduces me to her daughter, Liya, who looks to be about fourteen years old, but who grabbed my luggage with a vigor that I did not dare challenge. We navigated our way through a sunbaked obstacle course of solicitous taxi drivers who make their pitches to me as though Mary and Liya were invisible and who themselves maneuvered so nimbly they may as well have been. It was a relief to finally close the passenger side door of Mary's small Toyota behind me, even though we had to tempt fate and quickly open all of the windows in the name of aeration.

"Mary, thank you so much for picking me up. I really hope it did not disrupt your day too much."

"Doctor, if you come from as far as you did, how could I not?"

"Please, you need not call me Doctor unless you prefer I call you the same?" She responded with a wave that led me to drop it.

We pass out of the gates of the airport and onto what I took to be a local one-lane highway, passing an endless scene of thatch roofed houses that seemed to have been poured out in bulk onto the vast fields from some heavenly sack, with some rolling to a safe stop just at the edge of the road. A few, however, are nearly burnt to the ground, no doubt the scars of war. Women crouched over fires, cooking. Livestock roamed and gave the car a knowing look as yet another do-gooder arrived. I wanted to ask them to tell me how my trip would turn out.

"We must get you something to eat."

A few quiet minutes later, we suddenly veered off the highway, but this was not about a restaurant or her driving. Mary got out of the car and went up to a bare-shirted man sitting in the dirt, scraggly arms hanging over bent knees. I watch her wag her finger at him and nearly stomp her feet. But he gave her a dose of her own medicine and waved her off. Mary came storming back to the passenger side of the car, flummoxed.

"Doctor, you must come at once. I am sorry to bother you after your long flight, but help is needed. Please, will you?" This was part entreaty and part conscription, as Mary was opening my door before she had even finished. Liya also got out but opted to sit on the hood of the car and play with a yo-yo.

We walked back silently to the man, who was now fully prostrate on the ground, a raggedy baseball cap placed over his face and hands cupped behind his head.

"Malike, this doctor is here all the way from America. Now, show him some respect."

The cap comes off of his face. "Hello, sir."

"Nice to meet you. What can I do for you?"

"Ask Doc Mary," Malike hissed. Then he replaced the cap on his face.

Something told me that Mary was contemplating tearing the cap from his face but instead she turned and made her case to me.

Malike was one of her wayward patients and had schizophrenia. He had gone AWOL from the psychiatric hospital where she was the director. No medication, who knows what nourishment, and surely no bathing in about three weeks. In America, "eloping" from a psychiatric hospital was not easy to do, and when it happened, usually was met with what could often be an army of people seeking the patient's return—concerned family, case managers, and often the police. Although I had yet to see Mary's hospital, if it was anything like what you find in most of the developing world, it could be days or longer before anyone even noticed Malike was missing. As for outreach, families could be unreachable because they shun the psychiatrically ill family members, with stigma being thicker than blood; there are likely no funds for case managers; and police would likely just beat and arrest the itinerant soul. And there was certainly no cold weather to chase Malike back.

But there we were doing the outreach ourselves. Mary had been urging Malike to get into the car with us so she could take him back to the hospital herself and now hoped I could make a better case. I felt like a sham and not the all-knowing psychiatric expert she had invited to help make things better in her country (that's the answer as to why I am here). I cannot say I had ever done a roadside rescue in my years of practice and could not recall ever making more than two or three house-calls. I had special teams to do that for me while I played the puppet master from my office.

And I did not want to travel in the same car with Malike.

"Malike, why don't you come in the car and help Doctor Juma give me a tour? I just arrived from America and have never been here before."

It's a trick.

"You just heard the doctor tell me you had been at the psychiatric hospital. What psychiatric problem were they helping you with?"

They are the problem.

"Why don't you give them another chance; they want to help you?"

No, dey don't, man.

Mary walked off during my monologue and came back with a vial and a needle.

"Malike, if we cannot bring you to the hospital, we can bring the hospital to you. Sit up and pull down your pants."

The cap glided sideways to reveal an eye. Then Malike bounced to his feet and turned in one astoundingly balletic motion and ran into the field with the speed of an unheralded track star. This brought Liya to life, who ran over to us and offered, nearly begged, to run after him. Mary gave her a universal mother look, and we all lumbered back to the car. I could not tell if I was feeling more jetlagged or demoralized.

By the time we did finally get around to eating at a roadside food stand I decided it was jetlag. As we sat at a picnic table eating flatbread and peanut butter soup in post-Malike silence, my mind felt as though it had decided to flee its duties only to get as far as gripping the top of my head. Thankfully my stomach had remained at its post, and I managed to eat with instinctual gusto enough to reward Mary's hospitality.

I finally coaxed my mind down from the ledge so we could make the most of our time here. Not all psychiatrists like awkward silence.

"So, Mary, how did you get into the psychiatric business?" Am I sounding too much like a psychiatrist myself?

"Ah… probably no different than your reasons, Doctor."

I decided not to accept that. In my city back home, psychiatrists are as common as parking meters; here they are as uncommon as parking meters.

"Mary, maybe we had similar reasons, but I really doubt we had similar paths." My shrinky nudge paid off….

"Well, Doctor… I went to medical school right here in my country. There's no psychiatry in that. My professors never gave it a thought, nor did I. In the U.S. of A you get psychiatry, yah?"

In something of a trance, I nearly responded with my own yah. "We do. I think most medical schools are like mine, offering a classroom course in psychiatry and then a month-long rotation on a psychiatric unit."

"Well, Doctor, my… rotation happened during the virus," with a hint of sarcasm to underline 'rotation' for me. "I have been working for the Ministry of Health as a Medical Officer since the day I finished my internship. They used to send me where they like, but I mostly worked here in the capital city as a general practitioner. Lots of high blood pressure, diabetes, and the occasional tattoo from a marital spat. Used to be lots of HIV, but we got that under control long ago, you know.

"When the virus arrived in the land like the 11th plague there were bodies in the street, and I went to work every day wondering whether I would come home. I started doing home visits because people were too sick to come to us, and anyone who wasn't feeling sick was too scared. Then the boss reassigned me to the Treatment Units, where the ones lucky enough to get there hoped they were lucky enough to leave.

"You know, it was dreadful... they were locked up in these containers. It was hot, and there was no letting them out for air. No visitors. And no way to talk with their families. You know they took away all of their belongings and burnt them when they got there—including their cell phones. People here may not seem like they have much, but everyone's got a phone. The only visitors they got were us in our spacesuits come to check on them, give them their medicine, bring them food if they were in eating condition.

"I saw the toll this took on their spirit. And I knew that their spirit was about as important as the fancy medicine from the World Health Organization. So, instead of getting in and out as quickly as I could, I would stay and talk to them. I spent more time with them than I ever could with my sixty clinic patients a day, and I saw the power of listening. I started to read about Mental Health First Aid and how to provide support through psychotherapy—what's that called again?"

"You mean supportive psychotherapy?"

"Yah, there you go. I also saw how, when they got well enough to do more than lie there that they need something to do—books, playing cards to play solitaire, checkers to play with staff who would brave it, and even a radio if we could find one. I organized a donation campaign. Anyway, word got out about what I was doing. The nurses started calling me Mental Mary.

"Well, it all ended—thank the dear Lord in Heaven. But among the lives he took was the director of the psychiatric hospital. He was the only psychiatrist in the land. The chief medical officer for the Ministry of Health called me himself. 'Mary—I hear you found your calling.' Three years later, I am still the director. No psychiatry training, you know?"

And yes, that's what I am doing here. Mental Mary was going mental tending to the mental health gap in her country so big it was swallowing her up, and I am on what we call a needs assessment trip, trying to see how (never if) we can help bridge that gap between the mental health needs and help and throw a lifeline to Mary while we are at it.

Before she dropped me off at the hotel, she filled in more of her story, explaining how people would come up to her seeking her help in the grocery store and her home. Psychiatrists are big on "setting boundaries" with their patients, but that there was no room for that here. Everyone knew everyone, and even without a public transportation system, no distance was too far to go see the expert. I admit that hearing her story made me think that "boundaries" were just another American luxury, a way for us back home to end our workday in time to get to the theatre. It has also always seemed to me that America was founded with a view to distancing ourselves from tyrannical kings across the ocean and that as Americans migrated westward across the new continent settling their own parcels of land they went ever further and began distancing from one another. I do wonder if our affinity for boundary setting may well take off from that, as much a matter of culture as psychiatric technique.

But Mary did point out one boundary that worked in her favor. During the civil war, both sides left the psychiatric hospital alone, allowing her to move her family there for safety. "Those fighters were too scared of it."

I am not sure how Mary found our program or me, but I guess I am already helping—the number of psychiatrists in the country already increased by 100%. For a month. My thoughts are racing in the second wind that has come over me, strategizing as to where I should start. In its currents, my doubt gives way to big dreams. But then sleep conquers the superhero as my eyelids bring down the curtain.

Chapter 3

Berko

After they settled unto cushions on the floor, Londo bid the couple to begin with an outreached hand and a "Please…."

Hurt and concern raced neck and neck out of the woman's mouth: "My husband he not right. Been talking nonsense. Not even eating my cookin."

Londo pensively rested his chin in his hand and asked her how long it had been like this.

"Two months. We had to leave de town. We came because we heard about you."

Berko sat there half-spectating while Londo and his wife, Ife, talked about him. The details were lost on him, being stirred into the stew of thoughts and emotions that were his churning mind. It was a stew that could not simmer long enough to get past its parts. Things were not connecting, and he was aware enough to find this bewildering. Berko tried with all of his mental might to find his bearings in it all, to find some line of thought, even just some coherent thoughts, to which he could hitch himself and restore logic. The problem was that the best footing he could access left him standing with one foot on bizarre and the other on terror.

I am hungry. The cat hit the white. What was dat? Brown spill. Red hot. Blue the sky. Sing a song sad. Go dat way. The way of the lost.

Unseen: Field Notes of a Global Psychiatrist
Craig L. Katz
Copyright © 2025 Jenny Stanford Publishing Pte. Ltd.
ISBN 978-981-5129-42-7 (Hardcover), 978-1-003-56767-7 (eBook)
www.jennystanford.com

I am tired. Split it, hit it, wit it, knit it, nit in the hair, bear it, wear it, share it. Head on fire. Fire me now but don't spill the water. I stand for myself, but please sit. It's a riff off of a raff. Ife goes my way, and I don't go. Ife go, Ife no, help. I am hungry, but I am sad. What is dis? I need help. I will close my eyes and rest. When I wake up it be good. I can't close my eyes. What I see scares me. Who is with me? Need to go to the bathroom, but who in it?

Who is this man Ife speaks wit? Doesn't he know she marry me? He will kill me if I sit here too long. How can get away? I can head for de door and swipe at some plants to slow him. But what about Ife? Will dey marry tonight? How can I stop it? I can kill her.... Hey man, what you be thinkin? She yo wife, she be good. She here to help you. No way, man, stop dis thinkin.... Hey, dey want to kill me. I be in da way. Dey planning it right here. Dey think I am dumb. I can hear you. I see you planning my murda.

Burger, bird, word. Da herd plays da hand. And I share da stars. Cars at bars. I need a car to get away. What if dey stole the gas? Spare dem dare lives if dey get me gas. I need gas!!! Hats I like, but cars do. I hang dis way, dat go dat way, and dat wind blows. Sing me song when I talk. Talk, talk, talk, talk, talk. Rock n roll, I can roll away. Be safe and be good. I know, if I stand dis way, I be OK.

With this, Berko began to sit up, imperceptibly at first, and barely more than that as he rose without even pushing off with his hands. It seemed like he was being inflated from below the floor, unfurling more than standing, with any and all motions being reactions to an unseen upward force. Berko's face was emotionless, his arms dropped to his sides, and his clothes smoothed themselves. When he finally reached full height, his right arm elevated to ninety degrees with outreached hand palm down as though last to inflate. Next, his head tilted all the way to the left, the motion ending as ear rested on shoulder. Then, it all just stopped, and Berko stood frozen.

Londo looked up with searching eyes. And with Berko's motions having interrupted her account but providing exhibit A, Ife resumed, "You see dat?! Dat what he been doin. He scare people. He no pay me attention. He just stand dere. He scare people.... He got da spirit, yes?"

Londo had stood up to reassert his authority and responded without pause, "I do think so, sister." Then he circled around Berko as much as the small space allowed, eyed him with a professorial air, and eventually asked without looking away from his subject, "What else he do?"

Ife was eager to add to the record. "Sir, he act scared. He talk scared. He tell me da elder want him dead and try to poison him. So, he don't eat. I tell him I cook it—what's wrong with my food? Da elder have nuthin to do wit it. I ask if he wants me to cook new dings. He say he nobody's fool and dat I should not get with the elder on dis."

I am safe, woman. No eating now—I stay like dis, I don't need your food. You need me. You see me now and know I got power. Da lion got dat.

Londo wanted to know if he had threatened her. "No, but he say scary things. Dat's just it. He talk crazy or talk fear. Berko say he gotta go, but where? He even talks by self. Not pray and not to me."

You pray to me now. I am de idol in town. Put da food at my feet and go. "Go!"

Ife flinched and Londo seemed to jump right out of his sandals at Berko's roar. He stepped back and picked up the pace of questioning: "What he do now?"

You don't got to know. I got ya. You stand dere and get down. I da lord of all of you.

Ife explained, "He go quiet. But den I don't know. One night, he up all night yellin' nonsense. Dat's when de neighbors started talking. I keep him away from dem. I keep him home. My brodder came and tied him to bed. But den he yell like animal and people talk.

"De healer came to house. He said he de only way to help was to leave da house. He wanted to help de town, not Berko. He wanted us away, and de elder said it must be. We just married and dat our hometown. But dey treat us like outsider."

Outsider, besider, one-sider, insider. I de one , and dey know. Low down is the way. Dey afraid but sure ding should be. Pray to me—I will save. Oh, if it be. What do we? I do see , but you no. I am go wit it. Put 'em on with da tea. Pray. I judge. The court no go.

Londo wanted to know what he had been like when they married, and Ife explained that theirs was an arranged marriage approved by both parents and blessed by the priest. It all seemed right, especially coming on the heels of the end of the civil war. Berko worked for her father doing various chores around their family farm but mostly served as the driver. He picked up workers who lived far away and delivered bags of harvested rice to the big American company that bought and shipped it.

Berko and Ife had barely found a rhythm to married life when he fell silent. Ife loved the stories he told about America like they were his rather than the longshoremen's. But then Berko seemed to run out of stories, then words. Ife thought it was her fault until she awoke one night to find Berko cowering in a corner of their one-room home. He startled her with a loud "No!" when she pressed him to explain, and they both fell asleep crying, Ife strewn across the bed and Berko drooped in the corner. She was too afraid to bring it up the next morning, and Berko volunteered nothing.

In time, the storytelling revived like an angry spirit rising from the dead. American ships were transformed from radiant vessels to cleverly disguised pirate ships. Berko became certain that the rice bags he delivered had become weighted down by spy equipment. He would prove it to Ife if only the cameras would not catch him in the act of bag-ripping discovery. And most hurtful of all, Berko insisted that Ife's father was in on it all, seeking to prove he was a corrupt employee and unfaithful husband. Berko became so enraged by Ife's skepticism that she gave up trying to debunk this rubbish. Now she fell silent.

Ife was too loyal of a wife, and Berko too fearful of a son-in-law, to reveal Berko's suspicions to her father. But her father saw for himself. Berko talked evasively in words, maybe phrases, and certainly not sentences. He disappeared for unexplained hours with the company truck. He skulked around work and family. Ife's father accused Berko of drug use, but his son-in-law denied it with the matter-of-factness of someone explaining they care not for mango. It was her father who sent the healer to see Berko, and it was him who sent the healer away when he recommended that moving away was the solution. But when Ife had a miscarriage, her father confronted Berko's parents about being duped. But that just led to their having nothing further to do with Berko, Ife, or her family.

Ife's father told her to divorce him, but Ife would not truck this. She worried for Berko and what would happen to him. She had never wanted an arranged marriage, but it was not for her to decide. And Berko had grown on her as a good, devout man. Some husbands—

including her father—beat their wives. But not Berko. Men drank and got drunk, but Berko was inevitably in one of three places—home, work, or church. That also meant no drugs; she knew that was not his problem.

Ironically, drug dealers might have been the only people who would have had anything to do with Berko at that point. Merchants took to shooing him away. Parishioners at church would sit as far from him as possible. And their friends no longer came calling, which suited the suspicious Berko but devastated Ife.

Estranged from her in-laws, at odds with her parents, ostracized by neighbors, and all but evicted from their town, Ife took Berko and finally left. Her father gave them what would have been six months of Berko's salary, and they literally walked away from life as they had known it with that and four bags of belongings between them. Berko was making less and less sense at this point and talked about making a "pilgrimage" and "finding da path." Ife consoled herself that at least this all was making some sense to him and might for her someday.

Ife decided to visit her brother some 40-miles away. It took them two days and an overnight sleeping in the bush to walk there. Neither of them had ever been without a home, and she was terrified of being robbed in the night. But she was certain that Berko's ranting actually kept them safe from evil-doers, making her wonder if maybe he did have some newfound religious power.

They slept on two straw mats she had brought along, but Ife laid down in the dark dewy warmth well before Berko. He sat on his mat cross-legged with feet placed on opposing thigh and stared ahead. Ife had seen him do this once or twice before in the recent weeks and knew it to be associated with Eastern religions. Berko and Ife were Christian, and she had no idea where he had adopted this practice. At least it brought him some peace.

Berko was apparently not so lost in thought that he could overlook his sleepless wife lying next to him. He invited her to assume the same pose. In her easygoing way, Ife readily did so, figuring there must be something to it. The discomfort of the posture proved unsettling, but Berko's caring was the salve she needed. He kneeled directly behind her repeating softly, "It ok. We get dere soon. We get dere." Its rhythm soothed, and the breath of Berko's compassion propped up her back and her spirits. Berko still seemed to be in there somewhere.

When she asked to stop so she could sleep, Berko walked off and returned with an enormous coconut that he sliced open with his machete about one-fifth down its length. He and Ife both drank from it. He then sliced the remaining portion in half and carved out the intact side. Berko filled it with palm leaves he had ripped into one-inch slivers and placed it in between their mats, declaring, "We be safe now." And in her mind, Ife agreed and dozed off.

The next day Berko emptied the palm leaves from the shell and proceeded to place it on his head. It was irregular and did not quite span his head, but he "wore" it unflinchingly. That day, Berko spent nearly as much time righting it on his head as he did planting his feet on the ground one after the other. To passersby, he must have come across as someone stuck between doffing and donning. Ife shared her own perplexity with Berko and somehow felt reassured by his response—"It be, it go, we be, we go. Do and don't, but it will do. It got us." Ife acknowledged to Londo she had no idea why this made sense to her, let alone made sense enough that she could still quote it verbatim. But maybe it proved the dictum that it is not what is said but how it is said that matters, since she also recalled the ease with which her husband had spoken the words. It was like his mouth had been designed for them. Berko ultimately doffed, refilled and positioned the coconut shell on their second overnight outdoors, and sleep came readily that night.

Ife's brother would not allow them to stay in his house. He said his wife had health issues and could not tolerate the stress. They could sleep under the tree back behind their house and would be provided food until they figured out their next move, although her brother's tone made it clear to Ife that this offer was time-limited. Betrayals replaced dependability, and no path out of this nightmare proved itself. Meanwhile, Berko kept on announcing that they were right on target. Had he even become calmer?

Ife had no choice but to humble herself and her husband and accept her brother's "offer." She was seething but was clear eyed enough to keep it to herself. Her brother had a housekeeper who was kind to them, not only giving them meals but lending Ife an ear. She told Ife of a healer she had heard about on the other side of their county who was skilled at exorcism, but after her experience with her town's healer, Ife was not about to traverse the countryside for another.

Berko and Ife's stay with her brother proved especially short-lived, as Berko accused a fruit seller in the market of selling poison in the guise of purity, smashing several melons to the ground to make his point. When Berko announced he needed to seize evidence of the villainy and stormed off with a melon in each hand, Ife ran after him for fear of what he would do next. She meant to return and pay for the merchant's losses, but a police officer came after them before she could do so.

Berko seemed oblivious to the officer's demand for an explanation, instead thanking the office for his assistance and handing him the melons. Since Berko had so readily relinquished the melons, the officer may well have overlooked what happened and maybe things would have gone as well as they could. But Berko then demanded that the officer take them straight to the priest and when the befuddled officer told him that he would do no such thing, tried to grab the melons back. With that, the officer dropped them and then dropped Berko, pushing him to the ground and giving him a kick in the leg powered by years of soccer.

Berko was about to lunge up in self-defense when Ife inserted herself in between them like a referee. The officer cursed at her and began declaring how she was interfering with law enforcement; Berko cursed at the officer and began declaring how he was interfering with ways of the heaven. And as word gets out as quick as a group text message in villages like this one, Ife's brother arrived on the scene and, empowered by his standing in their community, pulled the officer aside and talked him down. Ife got her chance to pay the fruit seller, Berko avoided arrest, and the couple again found themselves exiled and heading only Berko knew where on foot.

Expediency decided that Ife should follow the housekeeper's advice after all and trek to see the healer of great repute even though it was a day's walk. When they got to Londo's village, it turned out to be home to one of the farm workers Berko had until recently driven to toil on his father-in-law's farm. The worker's mother offered them a place to stay for the night, but first they went straight to see Londo.

Berko had quietly deflated back into a sitting position in the course of Ife's narrative and seemed to inflate Londo in the process. Londo now had all the information he needed to declare his verdict—Berko was indeed possessed. He then declared his prescription—fasting for a week.

"It will starve the evil spirits to death."

Chapter 4

Sylvia

Sam felt relief as he arrived back home after visiting Londo. In that short journey, he concluded he had a lot to feel good about. He decided seeing Londo was going to help him, and tomorrow was Sunday, his day off. He was determined to help himself more by finally going back to church.

Sam's home was constructed, like most of the others in his town and his country, with cinder blocks. Gaps in the rows of blocks created windows, which were left open to the outside. A plank of wood served as the front door and more or less fit into the doorframe, as the door's roughly diagonal top and the horizontal doorframe created an upside-down triangular opening about an inch high at its vertical peak.

There was no doorknob, and Sam just pushed his way into his home. A business card wedged between the door and doorframe fluttered to the ground. Surprised, Sam picked it up and read with the aid of his eighth-grade education that someone named Molly from a group called Power Up had stopped by. It said something about helping tap the power of the community.

Riding his sudden buoyancy, Sam half-chuckled to himself that he wished he had power and wondered what it would be like to have electricity. His home was its usual dark self until his eyes adjusted

Unseen: Field Notes of a Global Psychiatrist
Craig L. Katz
Copyright © 2025 Jenny Stanford Publishing Pte. Ltd.
ISBN 978-981-5129-42-7 (Hardcover), 978-1-003-56767-7 (eBook)
www.jennystanford.com

enough to permit him to retrieve a candle and matches from a stack of three crates tied together into a makeshift cabinet. He rested the lit candle atop the lone piece of furniture in the room, a square wooden table with three chairs cut off what looked like the same wood. Otherwise, the light revealed a dirt floor and walls barren but for a foot-high wooden cross and a framed 5″ × 7″ photo hanging from a nail, showing Sam, his wife, and two kids posed in order of descending height. In one corner was a white metal stove under early attack from rust next to which squatted a propane gas tank that had been left unattached and unfilled for so long it managed to look despondent.

It did not take long for Sam to get his bearings in this 8′ × 10′ room, and after surveying his domain, he grabbed the candle and made his way through an open doorway into the other room of the house, the bedroom to the rear. A queen-sized inch thick mattress lay in the middle of the floor, and another one crumpled in half against the wall. Sam placed the candle on a three-out-of-four drawer dresser in one corner, where a bowl of water rested atop it from the morning. He splashed some on his face, toweled off with a musty kitchen towel that had "PRIDE" printed on it, and dropped his pants to the floor. The candle snuffed out, Sam plopped unto the sheetless mattress. He began to murmur a prayer to himself—"Holy Father dank you for dis blessed day and for de gifts you done have bestowed on me..."—but sleep assured that he got no further.

Sam awoke to the dogged bugle call of a rooster. Sunlight zipped through the house but not into his heart, as Sam's waking thought was a longing for his family. Loneliness filled the air, leaving him no choice but to inhale it like some poisonous gas. Sam felt paralyzed and knew his promise to attend church was a folly from the outset. In fact, he unflinchingly dismissed the value of prayer and silently conveyed to God that he would have to earn Sam's faith back if he wanted it.

Sam lay there awake for several hours alternately berating himself and berating God, albeit neither for any particular reason on this particular morning. The rooster had long since tired himself out with its optimism, but now Sam's mind darkly cackled away instead. A most uncommon occurrence finally silenced the brooding at once—a knock at the door.

Sam lay there wondering what to do, knowing of course what to do when someone knocks but feeling unequal to the task. He could not recall the last time someone stopped by, and in the interim, he had begun to feel like the people he heard got locked up alone in the treatment units during the virus. The visitor generously offered another knock, enabling Sam to gather his pants and reach the door in time to find a young woman, a young white woman, smiling at him.

"Sorry to trouble you, sir," she offered, "But my name is Molly, and I work for Power Up."

Sam's mind was alternately enjoying the rarity of sir-dom and remembering the business card in his door last night. "Hi."

After waiting an awkward moment too long for Sam to say more, Molly resumed. "I am from Power Up. Have you heard of us?"

"No, mam."

"Permit me to tell you about us, if I may. We focus on helping communities find their voice as individuals and a collective and implement change around that. I am one of our field coordinators, and I have been assigned to your town."

Sam looked quizzically at her, but before Molly could clarify, a bing emanated from her knapsack. *Why do I get a text now!!?* She took it off, rummaged around and silenced her phone without reading the message. After she zipped backed up, she resumed, "I should explain…." Now her knapsack buzzed, but she went on. "What I mean to say is that we help your community be as strong as it can be, to 'power up.'"

"What this means is I first need to get to know everyone I can in town and that includes you." Buzz.

Molly could no longer ignore her beehive of a knapsack and apologetically checked her text messages. There were three in a row that read, "Code Red." Molly went ashen. "I… I am sorry. I am going to have to go right now. An emergency. My apologies. May I come back?"

"Yes, mam, you can if you would."

Molly fished in her bag once more. "Many thanks. Here, here is a Power Up flashlight. It has rechargeable batteries that I can charge for you when I see you next… so you can start powering up in the meanwhile."

Sam stood in the doorway feeling even more confused and watched Molly scurry off.

"What's wrong?" Molly panted unceremoniously into the phone as soon as she got back to her car.

"Molly, your mother's no good again." It was their neighbor, Virginia, back in the small town where Molly grew up. This was not the kind of neighborly call you might expect in rural America in between church socials and block parties. It was a system they had worked out.

"Sylvia was up all last night tending her garden and landscaping. I probably would not have known a thing but for her ringing my bell at what must have been 3:00 am and asking me for a power saw so she could take one of the trees down...," Virginia narrated. "I told her, 'Sylvia, I don't think you should be doing this, at least not right now. Maybe get some rest, and we'll see what we can do in the morning.' She was all flushed and talking a mile a minute like she does when she gets this way. Like the very existence of earth as we knew it counted on her cutting down that tree."

"So, what happened?" Molly hoped the long-distance call would conceal her impatience, as she owed Virginia for making her mother her business.

"She stormed off saying I didn't understand. I wasn't sure what to do next and then I drifted off on the sofa with the phone in my hand wondering whether I needed to call the police. I just woke up with the sunrise and thought I should call you, and so here we are."

"So, it's around 6:00 am your time right now, I think. Where is she? " Molly realized that was as much a question of her mother's state of mind as it was her whereabouts, but she was counting on Virginia only for the latter.

"I don't know, Molly," Virginia confessed. "Her car is gone and all the lights in the house are on. I tried knocking just in case, but no answer."

Molly thanked Virginia and told her she would get back to her. Sylvia had manic depression, and Code Red meant Virginia suspected she was getting too high, too happy—manic. Code Blue would have meant depression—bad depression. Molly bought Virginia an international calling card to use when she needed to reach her about her mother, but they used these text messages in cases where she could not reach her on the phone or felt unsure of the time of day at Molly's field placement.

Despite realizing that the hours that had passed were more crucial than the minutes she delayed in checking her texts, Molly cursed herself for placing her asinine interview with Sam ahead of her mother. I am busy helping others to power up when my mother needs to power down.

These were the thoughts going through her mind as Molly dialed her mother's cellular phone and fruitlessly waited for her to pick up. Then she remembered that her mother had signed on to the Code Blue/Red system, too. She could always text Molly if she noticed herself slipping one way or the other. Molly wondered if texting Code Red to her mother would register and gave it a try. While waiting for a reply, she began sending her mother's primary care doctor, Dr. Harbin, an email. Without a psychiatrist for hundreds of miles around their small town, he had gamely undertaken Sylvia's psychiatric care.

Molly's phone finally rang, and her mother was on the other line loudly asking, "Darling whatever is the matter?"

"Mom, where are you!?"

"I am at the library." That was not expected. "I volunteered to help do some landscaping after all of the tax cuts." Her mother sounded out of breath. Sylvia herself had the presence of mind to know her thoughts were flying a million miles per minute and trying to make their way out of her mouth as fast they could. Thankfully or not, not all of them could.

I alone can do what they need here. They got the right person. Those bushes have to go. Or maybe I will cut them into topiaries. I like topiaries. I should have been a florist. Or a landscaper. Or maybe the mayor and then hire the right people to do this job for me. The morning sky is just beautiful. I should do this more often. Where's my camera so I can capture the moment? If I do all of this right, they will make me mayor. Or maybe I can just work on the mayor's house. After that, the White House is sure to follow.

"Mom, that's great, but it is 6:00 am in the morning. Why are you doing this now of all times?" At least she was not at a bar.

"Honey, don't some landscapers get going early in the morning?" In fact, Sylvia knew what she was intending to do was more than was asked of her and was best done stealthily. Having come to see the public library's grounds as her canvass, Sylvia assured herself that people did not always appreciate the work of an artist until later.

"Mom, have you been taking your medication?"

The question felt like a punch in the stomach—and from her own daughter! But it seemed to liberate her more rational self from the mental vortex. "Why dear, what does that have to do with anything? But if you must know, I did run out of my lithium about four days ago and just have been too busy to drive all the way to the pharmacy. I can pick it up if that will make you feel better."

"Mom, it really would make me feel better." Molly knew emphasizing that it would help her mother to feel better would be pointless since her mother felt great. "I am on another continent and constantly worry about you being all by yourself. Somehow you take the medicine, and I feel the benefit. That's how connected we are." She knew she was appealing to her mother's acutely outsized ego, but it was also in some sense true.

"Molly Katherine, the dear lord would have it no other way. We are bound together in love and peace, and our souls are like one.... Forgive me my busy little head, they are one. If taking my medicine will cure what ails you, I am blessed to be able to do that as a mother. Not all mothers or daughters are so lucky." Sylvia somehow knew to keep the next thought to herself—that God, Molly, and herself were a holy trinity whose very existence can heal all who ail. This inspiration was at that point not in the mainstream of her thoughts but making its way in from the margins. Her master plans for the library felt cosmic enough.

At that point, their call was blotted out by a loud noise that Molly eventually realized was a siren on her mother's end. It stopped suddenly, replaced by rustling and whishing sounds. When it finally turned silent, there was no response when she asked her mother what was happening. Then a beep-beep-beeping sound officiously declared that their connection had been lost.

Molly tried deep breathing to calm herself as she tried to call back over and over. In between these calls she sent up a flare to Virginia via text, "Mom is at the public library. Can you go??"

Finally, a phone call from her mother came through even as Molly dialed, "Honey? The police officer would like to speak to you."

She hoped that one of the veteran officers who knew her and her mother would get on, but they had all since retired. Instead, someone sounding like a boy got on, "This is Officer Regents. Are ya Ms. Sylvia's daughter?" When Molly confirmed her identity, he went on, "We have a situation and need ya to meet us at the present." Molly had been away so long she had to think a moment to figure out he meant "precinct."

Molly's heart dropped so far it nearly reached home. Her nightmare had come true—she was needed at home but was helplessly across the world. She conveyed her whereabouts and then explained, "My mother has manic depression and stopped her medications. Our family friend is on the way to the library. Please, sir, can you wait for her?"

"Manic depression, miss? Shouldn't yur muther be in an institution and not running around out here? Do ya know what she did?"

I don't want to know. "No, officer—please tell me, sir."

Officer Regent sounded like he had been rehearsing for this moment as he instantly began, "Well, it seems like ya muther got it in her head to fix up our little library here in town. Got so eager she couldn't sleep and came down here loaded for bear with hedge clippers, a shovel, her perty little gardenin' gloves. And her pink pajamas....

"I am not so shur what exactly she had in mind except to say somethin' about making it 'a library worthy of a king.' Her grand plans musta included a pool worthy of a king, as she left the library's lawn hose on so long it sent water cascading into the Reddy's backyard just back a' the library. Their property is carved out of that hill down below, and the water done gone plunging down the wall of stacked railroad ties into their backyard like a waterfall. She must have been running that water for a long while.

"Anyway, would be perty to look at 'cept it then seeped into their living room. Their dog is a good one—he just barked and barked at this lil' home invasion until they woke up. The confused Mr. Reddy came out and asked ya muther to pleeze shut the water, at which time she told him no way ya stop an orchestra midway through them their performance. When Mr. Reddy did try to walk toward the hose to shut it off, she stepped in front of him with her clippers and told him to scram. Hmmm…. Scram he did and called us."

Officer Regent paused with an air of accomplishment and some hope that a question from Molly would permit him a storytelling encore. But then, just like that he asked "Ms. Sylvia Junior" to hold on and excused himself. Molly was left to her thoughts and her greatest fears, including that her mother would wind up in jail today. She was cursing her mother in between cursing herself when Virginia's voice came on the line.

"Molly? It's Virginia. It's going to be okay. I spoke to the officers and explained things. They say that Sylvia has to come with them to the precinct but won't be arrested. They want her to wait there until she can see Dr. Harbin. Turns out he once helped the younger one's cousin. Must have done a good job."

Molly replied with a strange mix of gratitude and bother, "That sounds great, Virginia, but how are we going to get her to see him? Will she go? I mean, does she get this?"

Virginia conceded, "Well, I thought you better talk to her about this. Sylvia!"

After some more ruffling, Sylvia spoke demurely into the phone, "Hello, my dear. What's happening?"

Molly nearly roared, "Mom, what's happening is you nearly got yourself arrested. And if you do not see Dr. Harbin today, you will be. Do you understand?"

"But what does Dr. Harbin have to do with this?" Sylvia queried. I just go to him and talk, talk, talk and he just listens, listens, listens. Waves his pen like a wand and the very cure of me. It's like he is some sort of a guru or magician, except he's not.

"Mom! Your lithium, you need to be back on your lithium."

That statement went clang in Sylvia's mind, like it rang an unseen bell. Her speech was slower as she responded, "My lithium, yes of course. You were just beginning to remind me about this matter when the kind officers showed up. Do I need to see him today? Can it wait?"

"No, mom, it cannot. Virginia and I are going to arrange the appointment and you are going to do nothing but wait at the precinct until your appointment. OK?

"Yes, Molly, it's okay...," she replied in defeat.

"Mom, Virginia will get you some breakfast and a change of clothes. I love you mom."

Virginia got back on, and they worked out a plan for her to leave a message with Dr. Harbin's office and then help feed and clothe Sylvia. Molly tapped out an email (Subject: Code Red!!!) to Dr. Harbin even as she spoke, apprising him of the situation and telling him to expect a call from Virginia. She concluded it by writing, "Thank you for being there even though I am not."

Molly reminded Virginia to use some of the cash she left with her to buy the breakfast, including for herself. She ended by asking to speak to Officer Regent one more time to assure herself that he had bought into the plan. He had, although he signed off with this conclusion: " She is a crazy one she is. She done wind up in the loony bin if she ain't careful."

Molly was left staring at her phone—an image of a daughter at a loss. If could well earn a place in a textbook with the caption, "Global mental health is not just international health." The accompanying text would acknowledge that there is a longstanding tension in global health of all kinds between choosing to help out overseas and helping out at home. There are hundreds of communities across every state in the U.S. that are designated by the federal government as mental health shortage areas due to lack of mental health providers. But most such places probably still have far more resources than most of the developing world. And the calculus as to who merits the attention of mental health professionals more among domestic communities and then between domestic and international communities rides on rough ethical seas. In a world of vast unmet mental health needs and not-so-vast resources, it sometimes simply comes down to who asks for help—like Doctor Juma.

Chapter 5

Sam II

A second knock on the door in just days was so crisp that concern for the four walls darted through Sam's curiosity for who or what was on their other side.

It was the return of Molly.

"Hi there, remember me from the other day? Molly from Power Up…. Powerrrrr Up!" she cheered in 1-2 unison with a thumb up, arm up.

Sam wobbled from the pulse of energy. "Good afternoon, madam. It's real nice to see you."

"I am sooo sorry about the other day. Hey, how's that flashlight?"

"Yes, mam… it much appreciated." Sam could not remember where he put it, and his mind could not possibly accelerate enough to reach the answer before she asked if it needed recharging. Instead, his search halted as he warned himself, " Remember your ways are in full view of de good Lord," and he admitted he had lost it.

Molly took off her sunglasses as though to get a closer look at Sam and said, "My friend, you look like you need to be re-charged…. Hey, excuse my rudeness. What's your name?"

"Sam… Sam Ervil Gaye."

"Nice to meet you, Sam. May I sit down?"

Unseen: Field Notes of a Global Psychiatrist
Craig L. Katz
Copyright © 2025 Jenny Stanford Publishing Pte. Ltd.
ISBN 978-981-5129-42-7 (Hardcover), 978-1-003-56767-7 (eBook)
www.jennystanford.com

They sat in two chairs Sam brought out and propped against the house, both facing the street while catching some shade from the jagged overreach of the tin roof.

Molly explained that Power Up was a non-governmental organization that works to empower the voice of communities, enabling them to take charge of their future instead of waiting for "top-down solutions" to things. She passed another flashlight to him and explained that it symbolized the power of the people.

Sam flinched at this, as his mind found the wherewithal to begin racing, mostly incoherently but with at least one coherent thought: I can't fight again.

When the virus had wrought its devastation and containment efforts finally began to turn back the tide several years ago, a different virulence took hold of the country. Leaders of the majority ethnic group of the country began pointing weather-beaten fingers at the wealthier minority group. They stoked fears among the more rural, poorly educated majority that the virus had been a curse placed upon them by the upper-class ethnics. There was no evidence whatsoever that the virus took sides, nor was any motive ever proffered for why they would do such a thing, but it did not matter.

Long-simmering ethnic and class resentments exploded, like so many matches struck along the beams of the drilling rigs operated by the majority on the minority-owned oil fields. The social structure of the oil fields in fact came to define the sides of the war to come. Oil magnates, who sometimes acted more like warlords, had long been slangily known as "Buzzards," capturing both their penchant for descending bird-like on the oil fields in their helicopters and the predation experienced by their workers. Once the allegations about the virus caught on, all members of the minority class became known as Buzzards. Da People suddenly became the Bustards, a much more earthbound and conflict-averse bird. It was Da Buzzards vs. Da Bustards.

Sam, his wife, and their families were members of neither ethnic group, which is why he did not have entry into the oil fields and was left to the much less remunerative work in rice farming. They were a minority and did not even merit a bird moniker.

"Maam, I can' t fight no more. I done dat."

"The war, Sam?"

"I wanted no part of it. My family ain't never got sick, and we don't point no fingers. The good Lord says to point at yourself. I admit my sins. What others do is de Lord's business."

"Some Bustards come knocking on my door—just like you but no battery light. At night, dey got torches. And any time of day, dey got machetes, dey got guns, dey got da devil in their eyes, too. Dey keep coming, and I keep quiet. I keep da wife and girls quiet. I don't know what dey want anyway. I no Buzzard—my home is smaller dan a Buzzard's bathroom. I got no bathroom."

"I could not hide forever. I had to go to work da field."

"I hear, 'Hey Sammy, good friend.' Dey say, 'You now a Bustard.' Dey smell like palm wine."

"I say, 'Hey, I ain't no Bustard before when I needed work. What dis now'?"

"Dey say, 'Ahhhh…. You know you always a Bustard, man.' I keep walkin."

"One, he lives on my street, he goes and runs right in front of me. Comes up to me, and he do say, 'You ain't a Bustard, den you a Buzzard.'"

"They all laugh de devil's laugh."

"I keep walkin'."

"But then dey circle around, and I can't leave. One I never seen before, he big and he walks right up to me and grabs me by de neck, like he can just pick me up off de ground dat way, and say, 'Break da birdie's neck'?"

"After dat, I had to go with dem every day."

"I am so sorry, Sam. I am sorry they did that, and I am sorry for it all."

They're staring ahead, and some children go running by, chasing a dog with sticks, their gaiety lightening the mood.

"Sam, I want you to know there's a way to fight that does not involve guns. You know that, right?"

"Yes, miss, I sure do. What do you get at?"

"Power Up—we want you to use your voice to fight, not your fists."

"What I fight for? Dose kids there, my kids used da play with dem. Dey be friends. Now what I got? What words bring dem back?"

"I am so sorry Sam for your loss. Did your wife die, too?"

"Die?" Sam shivered with emotion, his body seeming like it was on the verge of exploding out of his skin. Instead, he just exploded, "Who die?! Dey leave me! I die!!" Sam lunged into the dirt that is the roadway and stormed off, the flashlight tumbling off his lap to its own death in the process.

With her heart slamming hard into her chest as if to try to get out for a look at what exactly just happened, the surprised Molly let out the loudest "Hey Sam!" she could. Who knows if Sam even heard it as he never paused nor turned around. Molly did a few rounds of box breathing to relax herself like she learned to do in the face of her mother's explosions (inhale for four seconds, hold it for four seconds, exhale for four seconds, hold it for four seconds and pray that in 16 seconds you've managed to blow away your demons). Then she left a flyer on Sam's seat advertising a "Power Up meet-up" the following week and slinked away.

Sam did not come to the meet-up despite the otherwise very good turnout. Molly took attendance, and when compared to her outreach list, only one other "recipient" failed to show up for this first of a series meant to help the men of the town "find their collective voice." Such a rate of return would net her another "point of light" in her record toward admittance into the "Points of Light Honor Society," but Sam's absence left Molly no room for self-satisfaction. Failed outreaches are an occupational hazard, but for some reason Sam's stuck with her.

Molly went by Sam's home afterward and, opting not to knock on his door, dropped off another flyer advertising the next meeting. Sam did not show up again. This time Molly needed to enquire after him—has anyone seen Sam Gaye?

One voice rises up: "Ms. Molly, no one done see Sam dese days."

"What happened to him?"

"Dunno. Maybe de spirits got him. Or maybe he done got a girl somewhere." Collective laughter replaces the collective voice.

Afterward, another gentleman comes up to her. "Ms. Molly, I don't think Sam been gone anywhere. No, mam. I don't think dat boy ever leaves his house."

This time when she went back to Sam's home, Molly knocked anew. There was no answer and no visible light inside. Emboldened by one of those ubiquitous flashlights, Molly opted to let herself in. Since most homes here only get padlocked from the outside when the homeowner goes out, the absence of a lock was a pretty good sign it was occupied. She found Sam sleeping on the floor of the front room, two empty jugs of what she knew were the reusable type usually reserved for palm wine on the floor. Having come this far and feeling like a burglar, Molly now had no idea what to do next, and hoping he was just drunk, she left, forgetting to leave another meeting notice.

At that point, Molly was only coming to the town weekly for the Power Up meet-ups, and one night, after what must have been the fifth or sixth meeting, she saw Sam sitting in a solitary chair in front of his home, as though she had imagined his flight and he had been sitting there all along.

"Hi, Miss Molly," he mustered with a wave of the hand from an arm that seemed like it was tied down to the arm rest.

Her bus ride back to the capital could wait. "Sam, how are you?"

"Ms. Molly, I did get your invitations, and I dank you. No disrespect in not showing up, ya know?"

"I know Sam, but what's going on?"

"I just so tired, maam. So tired. Got no energy. You know, you right you were when you said I needed to be charged. So right...."

Molly sat on the ground at Sam's feet. Remember they told us to use body positioning to help level the playing field with our recipients.

The usually gentlemanly Sam did not get her a chair.

"Sam, do you remember when we last met and..."

Sam interrupted, "I do apologize for dat, oh I do. How do they say it in the States... you tripped my nerve...?"

"I think you mean I stepped on your nerves. Something I said hurt you here, like here in your heart."

A single, lonely, tear quietly descended down Sam's face. It clung to the jawline and then dove into oblivion, a performance heralding the story to come. Sam stood up in soliloquy, gazing half skyward as he spoke.

"Amara, my lady, she don't want me to join the Bustards. 'Sammy, you're not one of dem. You no fighter. We be better than dat.'

"I tried to explain to her dat I had no choice, but she said the good Lord always gives us a chance to choose what's good and right. I told her if I do what's right it will be de last thing I do."

"I promised I won't hurt anyone. I lay low in our gang. We go out every day roaming de streets, looking for Buzzards. If we don't find 'em, we find their homes, their offices. Then we find 'em. As things got bad, we had to search 'em out more and more."

"When we find them, we hurt them bad, sometimes just leave 'em to die. I dink they were too afraid to kill 'em all de way. The boss man, he liked to finish 'em just to the edge of meeting their maker and say, 'OK, let's leave this Buzzard for a vulture.'"

"I stayed back. I never hurt anyone. I dink no one noticed, but den someone I called Little Boss Man 'cause he was second in charge, said, 'Hey dere Sam, training's over. Time to get to work. De next day dey push me to the front, looking at this pathetic Buzzard tied in his chair and handed me a machete. Dey had me do what none of 'em could do. I finished him off. Never done that before.... Not most of dem done dat either...."

Sam seemed to collapse into his chair. What she dink of me now?

Molly felt paralyzed. What am I supposed to say?

"Well, after that I keep dinking of de poor Buzzard and I can't stop. But palm wine—I figured out why all of 'em Bustards smelled of it. It done make it better. Drink and you no dink. Amara, she don't like it one bit. 'Now dey have you drinkin'. Is that part of de job? You no good like dat. What kind of pa are you to da girls like dat?'"

"I wanted to tell her why I drink like dat. But I knew I done break my promise. If I told her what I did to that man, den what? But da problem is I could not stop drinkin' else I start dinkin and because of dat... dat..., she done gone and leave me. She took my two girls and went straight to de other side of da country to her ma and pa."

"After da typhoon and da fighting stopped, I did stop, too. Most of de time no more palm wine. But it done do my body no good. Must have damaged me. I just don't feel better. I went to Londo, the healer, and he do dis and dat but still I feel dis way."

Molly finally felt like she could say something that would not risk hurting Sam more, asking him why Amara had not returned.

"I don't know, Miss Molly. Amara don't take me calls—she don't even know I gone and stopped. She don't know a ding but what she dinks. And my girls…? I am bad. Dey probably better off dis way. But I am not."

Molly tried to find her footing, to find something she can do. Power Up meet-ups were not what he needed right now. "Sam, you need to see a doctor."

"Yes, maam, but no doctor here. Just Londo. No doctors anywhere around here."

"Sam, you must come to the big city, to the capital. The hospital there has doctors, some of them even went to school in America."

"Miss Molly, I got no money to go spending on that bus. I do send money to Amara—that she takes even if she don't take my calls."

Eureka! "Sam, I will give you money for the bus!"

Chapter 6

The General Hospital

The average person living in the developed world tends to hold one of two views of the average person living in the developing world—either biblically stoic in the face of their deprivations or counting the days before they can biblically journey for the better life of the developed world.

Sam's seatmate on the bus ride to the capital snoozed with head back in dental-chair pose while their chicken sidled unto Sam's lap. Bus-riding chickens were commonplace, but not welcomed, and Sam's strategically raised leg did little to redirect him for long. Sam had not taken such a long bus ride since before even the virus, and his seatmates left him especially down on its prospects. But Sam was not fantasizing about being on one of those shiny New York City buses he saw on a friend's television—he was wishing he were back in bed.

Sam's window seat did afford him fresher air and a view, and the pace of the bus spliced the window-framed scenes into a monotonous silent movie that mesmerized even if it did not entertain. He counted the number of kids that waved as the bus lumbered along like counting sheep at bedtime. The one action scene came when a pair

Unseen: Field Notes of a Global Psychiatrist
Craig L. Katz
Copyright © 2025 Jenny Stanford Publishing Pte. Ltd.
ISBN 978-981-5129-42-7 (Hardcover), 978-1-003-56767-7 (eBook)
www.jennystanford.com

of helmetless motorcyclists opted to take turns rappelling off the side of the bus with one hand creating a rhythmic soundtrack that went growl, thud, laugh; growl, thud, laugh; growl, thud, laugh. Still, but for a washed-out bridge from the typhoon that added an hour-long detour to the trip, it went almost as fast as the chicken could return to Sam's lap.

The bus let the passengers and chicken out at a nondescript intersection that was definitely more bus terminus than terminal, presumably designated by invisible signage only the bus driver was trained to read. Sam realized almost as soon as he stepped off into the urban cacophony that he had no idea how to get to the hospital, but the bus suddenly found its mojo and hurtled away in a puff of exhaust before he could ask the driver. But things were harder, and things were easier in Sam's country. Despite the din of the street and that of his mind, Sam somehow heard a motorcyclist shout, "Hey man, what you doing here?" Walter from grade school knew where the hospital was and without asking questions, zipped Sam off to see the doctor.

The hospital looked to need a doctor itself. Its earnest white façade had turned ashen from the smoke of war that not even the typhoon could wash off. On the other hand, the flood waters did have their way with the vast lawn, carving out an enormous pockmark of a crater. Walter decided to make the most of his detour by descending into and out of the depression and actually brought a youthful smile to Sam's face in the process. He left Sam off at the hospital steps.

Sam still looked lost as he stared up at the hospital entrance. It had long since been stripped of its once grand double doors for some counterintuitively martial purpose, and the empty doorway framed the building's dark interior so dramatically that Sam felt scared to enter the abyss. Seeing a doctor was an intimidating enough rarity, but what if he was about to put his trust in a white-coated spirit? Thoughts of Molly's spent money and his spent workday outweighed his fears, and in he went.

Sam's bearings were not much helped by the scattershot lighting of the labyrinthine halls, but a few pointed fingers later, he finally arrived at the clinic. It was at this point in the late morning standing room only. The ceiling fans were going through the motions, outdone by overheated and often feverish bodies that were like so many lit coals. And the clerk sitting at a desk seemed to be paced by the fans, as they languidly added Sam's name and complaint down with a look that conveyed doubts he would ever get seen, let alone get a seat. Sam did not expect any better than this but did hope he misread the clerk.

Two hours later he got a seat, two hours during which he would gladly have sat with two chickens on his lap. Still, he stoically bore standing even though fatigue was what drove him to come for help. Sitting was such a relief that Sam needed little else to pass the rest of the time, which was just as well since conversing with those around him was not an option. Even if Sam had any desire to talk, there was no conversation to be had unless everyone was speaking in coughs. Maybe they were all preoccupied with what ailed them. But there was no doubt also the smell of something else in the air—a newborn fear of strangers. Theirs had always been a culture known for its volubility, but the war led people to play their cards even closer than they used to in street-corner card games. Say the wrong thing to the wrong person and you were marked as a Buzzard, a lesson that outlasted the fighting.

Three hours later, Sam was called, and he bounded out of his hard-won seat. The long wait converted his uneasiness overseeing the doctor to a drive to do no less. His enthusiasm was not matched by his reception.

"How can I help you?" the doctor asked the paper he was taking notes on.

"Doc, I don't feel well. I am just tired."

The doctor looked up with an expression that said I-will-tell-you-what-tired-is and asked, "What else?"

"That's it, doc, I'm tired. It don't change. I sleep a lot. It don't go change."

"You got fevers, man?" No, sir.

"You got the shakes, chills?" No, sir.

"Cough?" No.

"Shortness of breath?" No.

"Stomach aches?" No.

"Diarrhea?" No.

"Vomiting?" No.

"Headaches?" No. But I am getting one now.

"You sleep with a malaria net?" No, sir.

"What's your name?" Sam Gaye.

"Sit down, Mr. Gaye. Over there." The doctor pointed toward an examination table. "Take off your shirt."

He examined Sam with newfound interest. Eyes, throat, neck, heart, lungs, abdomen, back, arms, hands. The doctor then opted to leave things above the waistline, steps back, and tells Sam he needs to check his blood. He pricked Sam's finger, placed the blood on a thumb-sized plastic cartridge, and then asked Sam to wait in the hallway. While obediently grabbing his shirt and heading for the door, Sam overheard the doctor pick up the phone and admit, "Next."

A frail woman hobbled up to the doctor's office and seeing Sam sitting just outside, pointed with her cane at the doorway and asked, "It's okay?" Sam didn't generally take himself to possess knowledge, let alone knowledge useful to others. For a moment, he even felt like his question had been taken away from him. But he gave her a "yeah," cocked his head sideways in the direction of the office, and then got lost in his thoughts.

Sam thought about how smart the doctor was and how lucky he was to be able to be able to see him. But could this be malaria? It did not feel dis way last time. Sam remembered how he felt like he was on fire and how his body would shake so much they thought he was possessed, a concern heightened by his level of confusion. Amara even called the priest to try to exorcise him of evil spirits. But if this was not malaria, then what? If that test says he's okay, what will the doctor do? Then Sam thought better of this line of thought and chastised himself for questioning the doctor. It's not for me to ask. De doctor, he decides.

A woman coming down the hall suddenly commanded Sam's attention. She was crying aloud and escorted by a grim looking nurse in full whites from cap to toe. The woman looked to be pregnant, but she kept howling, "My baby, oh lord my baby!" The nurse kept imploring over and over, "Now, miss, this is a hospital, please...." As they passed, the woman looked right at Sam and demanded of him, "Why me baby?!... Whyyyy?" Sam wished the nurse would answer her. He reflexively responded, "God bless you. God bless your baby," but his hushed words got lost in the maelstrom. She rumbled past trailing sorrow in her wake, having already left part of self somewhere further behind. So captivated was Sam that he did not even notice the slow-motion exit of the lady from her audience with the doctor.

"Mr. Gaye?" The doctor was ready to see him again, and Sam was readier than ever to see him, now at least as relieved to take refuge in his office as he was to receive the doctor's ministrations.

"Good news...."

The doctor explained that the malaria rapid test was negative, and that Sam had nothing to worry about. But Sam did have something to worry about.

"So, Doc, what's wrong wit me?"

"You need some vitamins, my friend. To get your strength back." The doctor wrote on a small pad of paper and gave the sheet to Sam with such verve that he may as well have said, "Voila!"

Sam clutched the prescription with two overpowering hands and looked down at it with a bent neck. Beholding this position of seeming veneration, the doctor was reminded of why he went to medical school, grateful for one of those special doctor-patient moments that keep you coming back. But a less invested observer might have seen resignation. The illiterate Sam was, in fact, trying hard to decipher the doctor and the paper, seeking a clue that could dispel his doubts. And in that sense, he was more or less praying. Dis say vitamins? Londo, he done say I need vitamins. So, he right... yeah? Yeah. He said he gave dem back to me. Maybe he gave wrong vitamins...? Maybe I need more...? Doctor now got it right....

The halls still echoed with the mother's wails as Sam made his way to the pharmacy. Anxieties ricocheted around his mind and into the power vacuum left by his punchless will, energizing his gait. And yet he was not fast enough. The pharmacy clerk notified Sam that they had just closed for the day, the open door notwithstanding. Without any sign of interest in the import of his prescription, she recommended, "Come back tomorrow."

"I don't live here. I got to catch my bus back home."

"Me, too."

"But I live in da bush. Got no money to come back tomorrow."

The clerk opted out of further dialogue and into a backdoor exit as Sam called after her ,"But Miss... Miss. I need my vitamins." What her problem?? After a minute of defeated silence, Sam slammed the counter.

A gentleman emerged from said exit like he were making a practiced entrance from offstage. Bow tied up in dress shirt and slacks with thick black eyeglasses angled up over his head and ready to descend into action, he filled the air with professionalism.

"How can I help you?" George the pharmacist said while reflexively reaching out for the prescription in Sam's hand.

"I need my vitamins. She said you closed, come back. I got no money to come back."

George engaged his eyeglasses and scrutinized the prescription, rubbing his chin in thought.

"Mr.... Gaye, I can try to help you." Vitamins again.

George knew the doctors often prescribed vitamins when they did not know what else to do. Lab testing was scarce due to broken equipment and shortages of reagents. And sometimes determination was in short supply, too, due to broken souls and a country-wide shortage of motivation. So, multivitamins could only help, giving the patients something for their effort and maybe even helping correct rampant nutritional deficiencies they lacked the equipment to quantify. But George knew he only had prenatal vitamins left, and he needed to save it for its intended use.

George asked, "Please permit me to call Dr. Ahmed," turned on his heels, and left Sam alone again.

Sam wondered who Dr. Ahmed was. His doctor had not introduced himself, and it took him a few seconds to make the connection. He glanced around the room while he waited, looking at white bottle after white bottle standing at attention and wondering what magic each held. Sam also could not help noticing all of the empty spaces on the shelves and wondering what medicine should have been there.

George had come back into the room and saw Sam's wonderment. "Yes, these are all of my little helpers. Couldn't do it with them!" He took a bottle off the shelf, emptied about two dozen oval pills into a new bottle, and affixed a handwritten label onto it that read, "Ferrous sulfate 325 mg. Take one per day on an empty stomach."

"Here you go, Mr. Gaye. Dr. Ahmed has prescribed iron to help strengthen your blood."

Sam admired the bottle in his hand and wondered whether he could ask questions. How much do I take? What it do? Would Londo approve?

He assumed all of the answers were on the label and was too ashamed to admit he could not read it.

"Do you have any questions for me, Mr. Gaye, before we do finally close for the day?"

"No, sir. I do dank you. May de Lord bless you and keep you."

Now, Sam needed to find his way out of the hospital and back to the bus. He did not even know when it would be departing. But he was feeling energized and free of worry, not even anticipating being back in his bed. Sam wondered if the medicine was so powerful it could already be working, although he'd never heard of such a thing. The bottle in his hand felt like a charm, but what he was feeling was neither pharmaceutical nor magical. George's can-do spirit had given Sam hope, replenishing what Dr. Ahmed had bled out of him.

Chapter 7

Into the Depths

No one asked me for identification, but it would have been redundant. My whiteness announced who I was or at least who people thought I was. Add in being a man and topping off the ensemble with my height, and I became beyond approach. I felt invisible even with all eyes on me as I emerged from my taxi and strode through the courtyard entry of the psychiatric hospital. It started to feel like a test of my ability to intuit my way toward Doc Mary's office, to witness my powers.

I looked around for a staff person, but I forgot that the absence of any demand that I produce I.D. was not just a V.I.P. exception but the way it was for anyone in most places where I have traveled. There were no I.D.s to guide me nor any helpful hints from uniforms or formal wear as to who were staff and who were patients. But then someone finally approached me.

"Hi."

"Hello, I'm looking for Doctor Juma."

"You a doctor?"

He led me in silence through a foreboding black gate to the immediate right of which was a conference room. There we found Dr. Juma sitting at the head of a rectangular table conducting morning rounds.

Unseen: Field Notes of a Global Psychiatrist
Craig L. Katz
Copyright © 2025 Jenny Stanford Publishing Pte. Ltd.
ISBN 978-981-5129-42-7 (Hardcover), 978-1-003-56767-7 (eBook)
www.jennystanford.com

"Ah, the good Doctor, welcome to our hospital."

Dr. Juma had everyone go around the room and introduce themselves—mostly nurses of varying responsibilities, including the head nurse, Nurse Providence, as well as some nurse assistants. Then they went right back to where they left off.

"So, Berko and his wife arrived here last night from where?"

One of the nurses explained that they had come from a county six hours away and that his wife, Ife, spent the night sleeping under a tree on the outskirts of the property.

"Well, sister, do go get her and get that poor girl some food the moment we're done, yah? Now, what's his condition?"

"He's psychotic, Dr. Juma. We had to give him a shot of haloperidol the moment he saw his wife leave. He's been sleeping off the antipsychotic ever since."

"Okay, please bring him to see me later. Now, who has a case for the Doctor?"

Morning rounds usually involve running through all patients with an eye to following up on urgent matters from the night before or anticipating those that are expected in the day ahead. More leisurely "case discussions" are usually reserved for afternoons, after the morning hubbub settles. But I had seen this before—interrupting the usual flow of things for the guests from the U.S. To this day, I am never sure if it reflects flexibility, expediency, or hospitality. I tend to fear it is the latter. Had this been inpatient morning rounds back at my hospital, the "guest," if they were even allowed to sit in due to privacy concerns, would likely be expected to sit quietly in awe.

Then there's silence as staff try to find something worthy of me to say. Finally, a nurse brought up Mr. Gibson, who's been "wanting to have his say." Nurse Willie explained that Mr. Gibson has been writing letters to the United Nations for weeks complaining of human rights abuses at the hospital. No one was exactly sure anyone at the U.N. was even receiving these, but what if they were? I could not tell how scared they were of that possibility, but I could tell they felt the moral weight of leaving his concerns unaddressed and were relieved to be able to offer me as an outside authority. He was said to have schizophrenia and needed to be repeatedly injected with sedating medications and even restrained. Dr. Juma had Mr. Gibson brought in and seated at the head of the table opposite her and to my discomfort at having to interview across such a literal and figurative distance, yielded her seat to me. A bulging folder that was his medical record was handed to me, but I thought it both discourteous and impossible to review it with the patient and my audience waiting.

I opened with a very routine "How are you?" But I might as well have waved a conductor's baton at an overeager orchestra. Mr. Gibson pounced with a cacophony of complaints held together by a sense of injustice and excellent, if affected, English.

"The police, they come to my house and drag me away, sir. No reason. I have rights. My parents just call, and they come. They're the criminals. They shouldn't have had me if they didn't want kids. Those police, they take me here in handcuffs. Off they come and then I get tied down. They just grab me. Last time my finger was broken, sir. No one helped me. I lay there like Christ on the cross. I miss dinner. They mock me, saying I am mentally ill to justify their depravity. They stick needles into me when they feel like it. I am no lab rat. Then they lock me in the prison cell. They do that to Nelson, to Faith. They do that to Eric. They abuse us. Why do they get away with this? Dr. Juma, she's the ringleader." A pause for a breath and a glare. "No way she can keep getting away with this. They treat us like animals in the bush. Do you know anyone at the U.N.?"

Before I could even consider my reply, Mr. Gibson rose from his seat and began goosestepping the length of the table toward me. I had no idea where this was about to go but found some comfort in my colleagues' seeming lack of concern. In the end, Mr. Gibson shook my hand, bowed his head, and exited the room stage-left.

I asked the staff for their reactions. One by one comments trickled out and gained momentum: "impossible patient," "didn't listen," "don't get the rules," "staff try real hard," "medicine don't work," "he don't take his medication," "why can't he listen?," "he's got no one to blame but himself," "he scares us," "next time the police should just keep him," "he attacked Johnny," "he threatens us."

It dawned on me that the staff may have sat so quietly around Mr. Gibson out of fear. When I explored more about his treatment, Mary said he was just on the antipsychotic medication haloperidol (aka Haldol), because they had run out of the other medication which had previously helped him, a mood stabilizer known as valproic acid that can treat the manic side of manic-depression. In fact, haloperidol and the anti-anxiety medicine diazepam (aka Valium) were the only medications they had in stock in the entire hospital for months. They were not sure if Mr. Gibson had schizophrenia, a psychotic illness, or manic-depression, a mood problem that at its worst can also create psychotic symptoms. But either way, valproic acid had been an important part of stabilizing Mr. Gibson while in hospital, or, at the least, haloperidol alone was not cutting it. Did I have any ideas for what else to do? I am as lost as you. Probably more lost.... I punted and explained I needed to learn more about the hospital and their resources before I could meaningfully offer any suggestions and promised the staff I would discuss this with Dr. Juma further.

Mary and I adjourned to her office afterward, where she told me more about the hospital. It was meant to accommodate 150 inpatients, but their census was usually around 200 patients. And patients usually stayed for months, even some for years. Even when patients got better, families often refused to pick them up or allow them home. Usually this was because they were afraid of or embarrassed by them. But she also suspected there was a financial component to some cases, since a hospitalized family member meant one less mouth to feed. Many of their patients were too disabled to work and contribute to their families, and their government did not offer disability income. Mary wished she could offer vocational training to these patients, but first she had to worry about when her next delivery of medications might come and what it would actually contain.

Sometimes the medications never came, and sometimes they would receive different medications than they needed or had become reliant on. Getting a supply of an antidepressant medication when she needed more of a given antipsychotic would invite a dilemma—just let their patients' medications run out or dispense the new medicine only because it was a "psychiatric" medication? Back home we have decision-trees from experts to help decide which antipsychotic or antidepressant medication to choose, but here they used whatever medicine fell from the tree. Mary admitted that she navigated the uncertainty of Mr. Gibson's diagnosis by leaning toward schizophrenia since they were able to count on having antipsychotic medications more than any other class of medications. When you have a hammer, everything is a nail.

I returned to Mr. Gibson's allegations of abuse, wondering whether she would have more to say in the privacy of our psychiatrist-to-psychiatrist tete-a-tete.

"Mr. Gibson don't realize we have the right to inject him with medication if he's out of control. You have that right back home, yah?"

"We do, although I think it is less of a right and more of a power. It often falls on deaf ears when we apprise patients of this. But we do make special lawyers available to patients if they feel they're being mistreated."

Mary clucks. "Hmmm. No special lawyers here. They need to trust us and should have all the reason on the good Lord's earth to believe in us. We're the only ones in this country who they can count on to see the humanity in them."

"He seems well-educated. Do you think Mr. Gibson is familiar with your mental hygiene laws?"

"Ahh, good Doctor, I am not sure that even I am familiar with those laws. I will tell you I could not find those laws if my life counted on it. Can't say I have ever seen them, yah?"

I suggested that it would be helpful for me to see them in order to be helpful with Mr. Gibson's situation. And I imagine it would be helpful for you and your staff, too. Mary just nodded and then asked, "Ready for your tour?" and got up. I started to join her, but she told me to wait while she got the head nurse, Nurse Providence.

Mary returned a few minutes later and explained that she never went into the hospital beyond the administrative offices at the entrance. Patients were brought to her office or the conference room. She added, "The hospital has its dangers, and if something happens to me, what happens to this hospital?" So, when Nurse Providence arrived, she was given two charges: Show me around and find a copy of the mental hygiene laws.

Nurse Providence started us off at the medical records room, which seemed like a higher-order version of medical records like Mr. Gibson's—bulging with charts instead of chart notes. It was wall-to-wall shelves of olive-colored folders in what must have been a 10′ × 10′ space, along with stacks of charts more or less defying gravity at the foot of the shelves. Nurse Providence clearly felt the need to explain that their medical records clerk was killed in the war, and the Ministry of Health had not yet replaced them, information punctuated by a skeptical twist of her head.

Next, we were off to the pharmacy. Where the file room was gorged with its contents, the pharmacy seemed starved. But it was organized nicely, and it did have the benefit of a pharmacist whom the fates had left alone. He had been sitting quietly on a stool reading a newspaper and was eager to show me around, opening the half-door to let me in. Bottles were proudly displayed on labeled white shelves like pieces in a museum. There were antibiotics, painkillers, and antidiarrheals. Although it's hard to imagine that you would have a hard time spotting psychiatric medications in a psychiatric hospital pharmacy, I knew from prior faux pas that it could embarrass the pharmacist to ask him. I found them only when I shifted my search to empty shelves. Shelf after shelf with labels such as "antidepressants" and "mood stabilizers" were empty, while on the antipsychotic shelf stood two large bottles of 5 mg haloperidol tablets along with vials of a long-acting version of the medication, known as haloperidol decanoate. On the "anti-anxiety" shelf were small vials of 5 mg/ml vials of diazepam for injections. I complimented the pharmacist on maintaining such a tip-top shop before we left.

Then came the center of it all, the patient area. I had seen better in some countries, but I am not sure I had seen worse. We stood in a large, windowless room rung by patient rooms around the periphery. The walls were an unfortunate gray that conveyed a sadness that the old building seemed to share with its inhabitants. And if they were any other color, it would have been hard to tell—the bare light bulbs in the ceiling fixtures were so dim they seemed to be absorbing, not emitting, light, in the name of survival. It felt suffocating even before a waft of sweat and urine overtook my senses.

Patients sat at picnic tables that offered some promise of good things to come. Some played cards, some were engaged in conversations, and some just sat alone, maybe over a drink or a snack. Patients sat on the floors, propped up against the wall, heads drooping here and there in a snooze. Patients milled around, like a sea of fish navigating to-and-fro. Somehow there seemed to be no tension as they glided past one another, even with one naked man among them. But I had no doubt I was catching them at a good moment. Indeed, Nurse Providence pointed out the padded seclusion room used to safely isolate agitated patients, where I peered through a small window in the heavy door to see a man in underwear sleeping on a mat—the quiet after a storm.

Patient after patient came up to Nurse Providence, but she deflected each away, moving past them like the big fish in the sea. She would say, "Now, Ms. Banda, I have a guest from America," and then they would look at me as though noticing me for the first time and turn on their heels (or were they flippers?) and float away. It made me wonder about the last time a staff person had talked *with* them rather than talked *at*, redirected, disciplined, or fed them. Maybe little was lost to interrupting morning rounds for me because the hospital was more of a desperate holding action than a therapeutic facility? After all, what could one psychiatrist do with 200 very sick patients? I asked about activities that you might expect in a psychiatric hospital such as art or music therapy, knowing that to go so far as asking about a staple such as group or even individual psychotherapy was simply not fair when I well knew the answer. Nurse Providence perked up as she reported that local churches sent volunteers who would play music, bring art supplies, or offer Bible study.

The patient rooms at least had some natural light, even if steel bars strangled the light on its way in. There was row after row of beds, in some cases side-to-side such that one could only politely enter the bed from its head or foot. Most beds were unmade, and many were occupied by sleeping patients. Mr. Gibson, though, was wide awake and was sitting astride a bed holding court with several patients sitting in a circle at his feet. He paused to salute me, a gesture I felt compelled to return.

We circled back to Mary's office, but she had apparently left for a meeting at the Ministry of Health. Nurse Providence asked me if there was anything more she could do for me, and I opted to proffer my business card with my email address so she could send me a copy of the mental health laws. Business cards are, of course, an efficient way to spell out my contact information and especially my name during my international travels, but it can feel like I am rubbing in my privilege when in a place where just finding a pen and paper to jot down the information is a luxury.

She then asked, "What do ya think, Doc?"

Oh boy.

What I saw was not only a lack of medication but a lack of much care. The very staff who were nowhere to be seen in the courtyard when I arrived were equally absent from the patient area. Were they all holed up in the conference room, as afraid as Doc Mary to be among their wards? Or were they laboring under what we might call in the lingo "learned helplessness," apathy born of a sense of futility? Dr. Juma, Nurse Providence, and the team were being asked to provide psychiatric care consisting of four walls, three meals a day, two medications, and one psychiatrist. I saw no psychotherapists, no social workers to engage and educate families, and for that matter, no families visiting loved ones. The staff surely cared but they were not able to care in the ways they were once taught to care.

What I said was, "You have an enormous responsibility here, and I can see your resources are not equal to your wishes for your patients."

"You said it, Doc. You said it. Thank you for caring. Would you like to join our mobile van tomorrow? We will be visiting our patients in the communities." Psychiatry outside of these grim walls? I eagerly accepted the invitation, and she promised I would be picked up at my hotel first thing the next morning.

Nurse Providence walked me back to the courtyard out front and left me to wait for my taxi. It felt like I had emerged from a cave. Half digesting my tour and half still taking it in, I counted several people sitting alone under the coolness of the trees and wondered who were the patients, who might have been staff, and who a devoted wife.

Chapter 8

Psychiatry in Motion

I needed a run. I went out the next morning before getting picked on by the sun and picked up by the mobile van. But my runner's high just never came as I navigated not so much the uneven surfaces and unfamiliar routes but the people walking and riding. Still, escaping collision was easier than escaping attention. It felt to me like everyone was looking at me—a white guy in skimpy clothes running from something unseen. I wanted to explain how my days are largely cerebral ones and how I need to open up the engine a bit. You are all on the road to get somewhere, but I am on it to get lost.

Past experience in the inevitably hot places we always seem to work lead me to leave plenty of time to cool off in my hotel room, but today my shower suffered from an unusual problem—only hot water! I was worried I would still be dripping hot when Nurse Providence arrived, beads of sweat telegraphing how I should just go back from where I came. I distracted myself by reading through the forty-one individually scanned attachments that were the forty-one individual pages of the law that Nurse Providence had emailed me last night with standout alacrity. In truth, I had never read through my own state's laws and doubt any of my colleagues ever did. On the other hand, these were translated into a "Patient Bill of Rights" that were posted throughout our hospital for both patients and clinicians to see. Even if it were posted at the hospital here, you would probably need a flashlight to read it.

Unseen: Field Notes of a Global Psychiatrist
Craig L. Katz
Copyright © 2025 Jenny Stanford Publishing Pte. Ltd.
ISBN 978-981-5129-42-7 (Hardcover), 978-1-003-56767-7 (eBook)
www.jennystanford.com

On page 17, it read, "Treatment may also be given to any patient without the patient's informed consent if a qualified mental health professional under the law determines it is necessary to prevent immediate harm to themselves or others." This certainly could speak to Mr. Gibson's concerns about being forcibly medicated, assuming the staff was administering this when his was indeed an emergency situation. But I could not verify that assumption nor know if they were first trying what we call "least restrictive alternatives" like talking calmly but firmly to prevent it from getting to that point without my spending more time at the psychiatric hospital, the necessity of which was clear but the prospect of which started my stomach churning as I thought back to what I saw behind those walls. I was feeling as helpless as the staff.

A text message heralded the arrival of the mobile van, and I ended my musings and bounded outside to find Nurse Providence sitting in the passenger side of a maroon van that announced itself it as "Ministry of Health—Mental Health Division" on one side, while the other side quoted the World Health Organization in declaring, "No Health Without Mental Health!" I have always loved that quote and thought it would have made the perfect bumper sticker if we had still used them. I believe bumper stickers went out of fashion due to concerns that they revealed too much information about the occupants of a car and were unsafe, but if only people were less secretive about their mental health, I do think the world would be a much better place. Of course, here most people do not have cars of their own, but there are billboards and T-shirts. In one storm-prone country, we made t-shirts for members of an alcohol self-help group who actually wanted to publicly declare their sobriety that read, "Alcohol can cause as much damage as a hurricane." Alcoholics not-anonymous.

A gentleman in a polo shirt with the Ministry logo on the shirt pocket stood astride the large sliding door of the van, waved me in, and closed it behind me. He turned out to be Johnny, a nurse assistant who was also our driver. After our good mornings, I got to learn about my companions, as I was always especially interested in knowing how people got into the psychiatry business in places where it was so marginalized. Johnny had been working at the psychiatric hospital for 15 years. He had always wanted to be a nurse but could not afford nursing school. Johnny never envisioned working at the psychiatric hospital because he admitted he never had thought about psychiatry or mental health for one second before a cousin who worked at the hospital as a cook urged him to apply for a job opening as an assistant.

I was seated alone in the rearmost of two rows of passenger seats, and in the front row sat Nurse Adanna and Angel. Nurse Adanna had been at the hospital for ten years, having begun working there right out of nursing school even though her classmates asked aloud if she was mentally ill for doing so. How did she go through with the choice even in the face of such peer pressure? Her father had killed himself when she was 13 years old, swallowing pesticide for reasons still unknown to her. Nurse Adanna's mother, teachers, and her priest all were on message in telling her that it was God's will and not for anyone to understand, but she was still trying. When she admitted she sometimes imagined a newly arrived patient could be her father finally getting help before it was too late, I felt weak and ashamed as I stared at the back of her head.

Angel was another nurse assistant who had only been working at the hospital for a year. She had taken refuge on the grounds of the hospital during the civil war and never left. She joked, "Well, Doc, I guess I am still waiting for Doc Mary to discharge me!" What has it been like? Much better than working as a cashier at the local supermarket. And anyway, it had been burned down during the war.

Somehow the quiet Nurse Providence's story felt off-limits, but she surprised me by volunteering for it.

Her youngest sister had become a patient at the hospital some twenty-five years ago while Nurse Providence was working in a public health clinic drowning in the AIDS epidemic. She was never the same after surviving cerebral malaria, seeing things and acting so bizarrely that the family had first tried taking her to a faith healer to perform an exorcism to no avail. Nurse Providence, as the only family who visited her and was not frightened of her, was so appalled by the care she received that she asked for a transfer to the psychiatric hospital. She and her sister were still there.

No one felt bold enough to inquire about my story, but I felt compelled to try to level the playing field: "Your stories are all more interesting than mine. Back home, there's a lot of support and a lot of options for going into psychiatry or any field of mental health. But you know, for a long while my grandmother told her friends I was going into neuropsychiatry because that sounded a lot more credible even though she had no idea at all what that was. And even my mother was concerned that I would become mentally ill by spending time around the mentally ill…. I will let you judge that for yourself."

Such raucous laughter and clapping rang out that it surely was audible to passersby out the open windows who could readily have taken it to be a rolling advertisement of the benefits of the mental health care we were peddling. Johnny suggested Nurse Adanna ready my injection, but she retorted that she could not spare his. This ignited an even louder round of applause. Then everything lapsed into silence that was interrupted only by hushed cell phone conversations and more of those ever-present motorcyclists toot-tooting their way around us. Soon, an overheated weave of silence, motion, and jetlag smothered me in a nap.

When I finally poked my head out from under that nap, not much had changed until we finally pulled over on a street corner on the outskirts of a small town. A few women were walking down the street with baskets perched on their heads, and a dog circled around nothing in particular. A nearby billboard with a United Nations logo in one corner proclaimed, "Buzzards and Bustards Flock Together!" And I just sat expectantly wondering what was happening as Nurse Adanna and Angel rifled through some of their materials and Johnny and Nurse Providence peered out the front windows, looking for something. I thought maybe we had gotten lost until Johnny pointed and yelled, "There!"

Nurse Adanna threw open the side door with gusto and yelled, "Come!" A scruffy man I had barely noticed in the streetscape squinted back and then approached us. The dog also ran over in canine anticipation.

"Good morning, Daniel," greeted Nurse Adanna, "It's very nice to see you. Roll up your sleeve."

An unspeaking Daniel walked right up to the edge of the van and did as he was told. The nurse took a syringe from Angel and popped it into his upper arm. Angel then passed along a brown bagged lunch for the nurse to give Daniel.

Nurse Adanna then concluded, "See you next time, Daniel. Remember the good Lord takes care of those who take care of themselves. Behave." With that Johnny checked off a clipboard, Daniel walked away, the door closed, Nurse Providence declared "next," and we drove off.

And that is how we spent the next few hours, repeating the process with forty-five patients in a mere half day, rolling up over and over with no fanfare, no discussion, and no evident planning. It was astounding. Yesterday's inaction turned into today's action, a transformation worthy of a superhero emerging from a phone booth. Somehow they knew where each of these patients could be found. For those patients out in public, they invariably knew exactly where they were with remarkable precision—a park, a field, a storefront. Sometimes townspeople saw the van roll up and without being asked, reflexively pointed the way to their sought-after neighbor. For the patients who were home, I could fathom neither how they knew they were home nor how they even found the home as not once did they look up an address. And that was just as well, as the towns were bereft of street signs and the homes of street numbers.

As for the actual exchange with the patients, they went off like a well-rehearsed ballet—short on dialogue and with an economy of movements. The staff remained in the van (honking when visiting patients' homes), and the patients ambled over and took up their place in the doorway duet. Only one patient refused to abandon a park swing, which is when I got to see Nurse Providence show her stuff, getting out of the van, swinging next to him, and walking him to the car with a hand around his shoulder.

That little was asked and little said is not how they taught it in medical or nursing school. Each of the patients was receiving the long-acting antipsychotic medication haloperidol I saw back at the hospital pharmacy, a medication that should stabilize them for about four weeks and help avoid "non-compliance" (an increasingly politically incorrect but still factually correct term for not taking medicine as prescribed). So, what was wrong with this scenario?

There was no doctor to review how the medication was going for the patients and to ask about benefits and side effects. There was no discussion of how their lives were going, no demonstrated curiosity about the person behind the illness. They were not even taking patients' blood pressure or other vitals, which I always took to be nursing 101. Finally, there was no evidence that a medical note was being written or would be written later about each encounter—Johnny's check marks were the only record of it, disregarding standard medical practice as I knew it but kindly sparing the overflowing hospital chart room. Even if they were to write a note, it would have been more perfunctory than even most notes are as so little was transacted or said.

All of this ensured the remarkable efficiency of the outreach, and no doubt was how the psychiatric staff did what they did with the little they had. I could not begrudge them that. It did seem they knew their patients, even asking here and there about their "mum" or other family member with a familiarity born of living in a close-knit community. There was certainly something very nurturing, if paternalistic, in going out into communities like this and in topping it all off with a lunch bag. I just could not decide whether I was witnessing something intimate or robotic. I thought about something a patient once said to me on a prior global health trip, a quote that has stuck with me not just in other countries but also my own—"There should be more counseling. Listen to our themes and not just talk about medication." Here they were not even talking about the medication.

Nurse Providence and staff never felt the need to narrate the trip for me, kindly admitting me into the inner circle of their mind-meld but overestimating my ability to tune into their wavelength. So, when we stopped the van for the 46th time and this time began getting out, I thought, actually hoped, we were stopping for lunch after a morning's work. It turned out we had one last mission—to retrieve Malike from his mother's home.

There was no need to knock on the front door. A government van pulling into a rural village and in front of your home drew plenty of attention. Kids interrupted their play to gather around in the dirt street in front of the house, as did a few cross-armed neighbors.

Malike's mother, wizened and intense, came out and straight off announced, "He not here," at which point I realized the neighbors were here to witness a duel.

Nurse Providence countered with good will, "Good day, Madam. Indeed, we are here looking for Malike and hoping to bring him back to the hospital. Have you seen him?"

"No, miss, I not see him. I not want to see him."

"Would you kindly call us if you should happen upon him?"

"I don't want him nowhere near 'til he see de pastor. He cursed, dat boy is. No need dat around here."

When Nurse Providence began to protest, Malike's mother turned around and began marching back into the house with a sprightliness that reminded me of Malike's sprint into the field. And then Nurse Providence pulled out her secret weapon. All but pushing me forward, she announced, "This doctor came all the way from the States to help. Won't you listen to him?"

Malike's mother stopped short of exiting the ring and turned back around, hands clasped prayerlike in front of her. "Good doctor, God bless you for comin' to help ma boy. Your mutha raised you good. I do see dat. But my boy need more blessin', not mo pills o' dem potions dey got."

"Maam, thank you for your kindness." Good start, and then I sputtered. "Your son has schizophrenia. It is an illness of the brain. Malike needs medication to correct his brain chemicals. He's not been cursed by anyone or anything except by his genetics."

Malike's mother reacted to my psych-speak as she should have. The part she understood clearly disregarded her beliefs and the part she did not might as well as have been said in a foreign language. Although I had no reason to doubt what Mary had told me about him, I had not myself evaluated Malike, and I think she smelled the deceit in my improvised attempt to live up to my billing. At the least, everyone beheld my hubris. Had I had my wits about me, I would have started out by asking her to explain to me about her son's possession (in private). After all, I have long been intrigued by faith healing. I was not even being true to myself or to the humility I preach to my students.

"Son, maybe you need a little mo' God. Yo mother done bring you to church, now look. You got to stand on mo' than dem doctor books of yours. Get yo Bible."

"Yes, mam. I do see what you mean." And then I slipped into kiss-ass, "Maybe I can come back sometime to read Bible with you?"

"Yah, sho. Just you don't bring dat boy with you. You see him, you done bring 'im straight to Pastor Louis." With that and a wave of her hand, she disappeared into her house. And all I could do was look back to the crowd, who seemed as disappointed as me that I could not beat the odds.

But what exactly was the contest anyway? My end of the mind-meld with the team led me to think the goal was to convince Malike's mother to let him back into her home when he next came around, with or without any exorcism. The mobile team could then reach Malike, whether with their injections and lunches or by hauling him back to the hospital. But my failure at debating her was a failure of debating her. Even my long-held conviction that psychiatry would be better for collaborating more with clergy seemed to suffer from my showmanship.

I read somewhere long ago that the "DSM," the American Psychiatric Association book that contains the criteria for every single psychiatric disorder and provides the basis for how we diagnose patients, all too often does not tell you where someone lives but rather their neighborhood (or, as I sometimes say of our often-imprecise diagnostic system, "patients' brains do not always read the book"). But in this case, falling back on it did not even get me to their country while Nurse Providence and Co. knew exactly where everyone lived. I bet they could even get to Sylvia, and it's entirely possible that Malike's pastor has a better beat on his soul than I do.

Besides opening up my eyes to a corner of the country's mental health services that was in good shape, my day with the mobile team revealed how quickly I can be thrust from wide-eyed back-bencher to starting quarterback. However much we all wanted me to be the all-knowing expert, I had to resist the call of wizardry. The answers to it all surely lie somewhere between what I know and what "they" know.

Chapter 9

Lecture

There exists an arc to that despairing feeling that strikes me every time I arrive in-country on a global mental health trip. I come to an inevitable inflection point where staring into the void gives way to a different existential threat—that of running out of time. My metamorphic disquiet probably hails from the fact that I, and most of my psychiatric colleagues, were not trained for work at the population level. Medical school taught us a systematic approach to diagnosing and beginning to address patients' problems, medical or psychiatric, and psychiatry residency honed our ability to diagnose their psychiatric problems and then taught us how to treat them.

But to evaluate and "treat" the mental health gap of any one community or country invites as much stress as it does excitement about figuring out how to make a difference on a larger scale. I can easily write a prescription for ninety tablets of an antidepressant (plus refills) for one of my patients, but there's no prescription pad big enough to conjure up 90,000,000 antidepressant tablets for a community that is home to mental health sufferers like all communities are. Instead, we have had to write the book on this in order to try to match our deeds with our will.

Unseen: Field Notes of a Global Psychiatrist
Craig L. Katz
Copyright © 2025 Jenny Stanford Publishing Pte. Ltd.
ISBN 978-981-5129-42-7 (Hardcover), 978-1-003-56767-7 (eBook)
www.jennystanford.com

Early in my globe-trotting days, I approached my trips in a stereotypically psychiatric fashion, taking things as they came and letting our host and country show us what they thought we needed to see and know. They usually do not have specific asks of us beyond helping them improve the state of mental health in their country, and implicitly, helping them feel less despondent about the prospects for doing so. I listened and let the patient do the talking. I have always said that the two most important things to know before going on any global health trip are who is picking you up at the airport and who you meet with to start your work on day one. They are shorthand respectively, for the unobjectionable if very shrinky concern for one's own sense of security and well-being and the belief that there's only so much pre-trip planning one can and should do from afar. This second point hails from a necessary respect for our host as the "expert" about their country and its needs.

But I learned that letting our partners "free associate" too much after getting past the introductions made for disorganized trips. They need me to show them how to best utilize my time in-country. I flew into one tropical city with but a week to organize a door-to-door mental health survey for my student team to conduct, but our host had not made arrangements for us to begin until four days into my limited stay. Instead, she still kindly took us on wonderful tours of the lush countryside. It's a good thing there were plenty of waterfalls to cool off in, as my mind was afire with frustration.

Eventually, one night on another trip when I was feeling lost staring down a country of millions of people trying to get past the trauma of two successive civil wars with the aid of one native psychiatrist, a framework for how we work with our host communities finally coalesced in my mind. I literally wrote the "Wheel of Global Mental Health" on the back of a napkin. It has us learn about "their" needs, their resources, and their will to bridge the two and to realistically ask of our psychiatric selves, the so-called collaborators, what our resources and will are to help them do so. And it's all arranged in a wheel because one change causes everything to shift (i.e., what do you do when a country literally runs out of psychiatric medications?). Here's what the wheel looks like on paper:

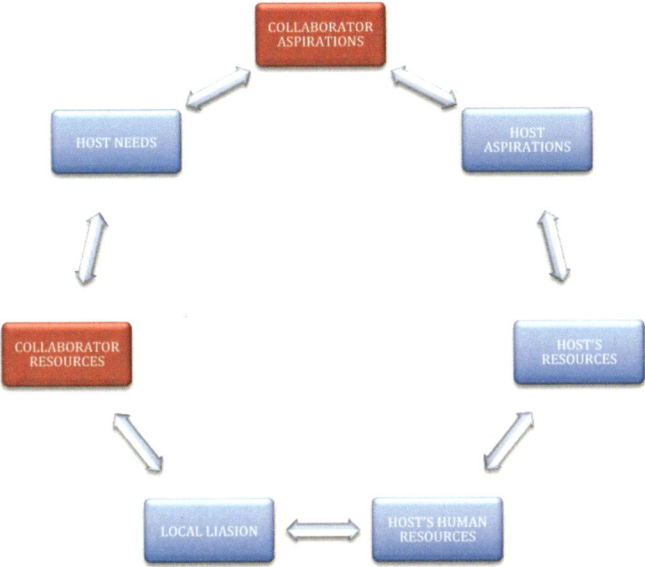

The wheel organizes global mental health projects between "we" (my program and I) as the Collaborator and "them" as the host. The host country or community suffers from a shortfall in mental health resources (human and other host resources such as medications) to meet its citizens' mental health needs (host needs). That's their mental health gap (= host needs minus human and other host resources). Someone there (local liaison) decides they would like to do something about it (host aspirations) and invites us to help. And the help we provide will derive from how much our expertise (collaborator aspirations) matches what the liaison envisions and how many resources my program can bring to bear on that meeting of the minds (collaborator resources). And if all then goes as planned, we will narrow the mental health gap, and in so doing, help people, communities, and possibly countries to function better and suffer less.

I do not have the resources to stock the shelves of a host's pharmacies with psychiatric medications or to staff their clinics and hospitals with psychiatrists or other mental health professionals to treat their patients in any way approaching sustainability. My program's main export is neither ourselves, nor our resources, nor even our money but instead lies in our knowledge. We teach, we train, we supervise, either improving upon the skill set of existing mental health professionals or trying to train new ones.

So, the part of the wheel we usually home in on is our host's human resources: Who can we recruit to the cause of mental health? A common answer—one with the full backing of the World Health Organization—is primary care providers. Because of how stigmatized mental health problems are in most places and how lonely it can be trying to minister to them in such a climate, we also provide an even more intangible service—inspiration for those who make mental health care their calling. Back home in academic medical centers like mine, there's so much teaching, training, and supervising that resident psychiatrists often complain it's too much. I should invite Dr. Juma to come to the U.S. to lecture to our residents about the opposite problem of having too little or none.

As for what the Wheel looks like in practice, it has been spinning since I met Malike along the way from the airport. It requires cramming the days with fact-finding opportunities about my "patient," the host, wherever I can. It's not exactly the comforting structure of a patient examination, but it at least affords a semi-structure around which to find one's way forward. After my visits to the psychiatric hospital and the mobile outreach van, I am already feeling pulled in too many directions and starting to get a gloomy feeling typical of most every global mental health trip when I inevitably start to question whether my efforts were worth the expensive airfare and royal treatment. The psychiatric hospital is a monstrosity that could occupy the resources of my program for many trips to come despite its tiny footprint. On the other hand, my experience with Malike's mother led me to want to explore the role of faith and other traditional healing practices in addressing mental health.

But there was still the broader healthcare system to consider. To really make a serious run at narrowing or eliminating the global mental health gap, so-called "non-specialists," i.e., non-mental health professionals, need to be on board with incorporating mental health care into what they do. I needed to see the public health system. Later in the evening after my post-mobile outreach musings, I asked Mary (yes, our local liaison) if I could meet with the chief medical officer of the Ministry of Health, which would be the senior physician in the public health system (the Minister of Health to whom they reported would be a layperson who was a political appointee).

Mary responded to the snap of my fingers the next morning in an apologetic text: The CMO was out of town. However, she followed that with a second text explaining that the director of the general hospital, considered the flagship of their health system and the biggest hospital in the capital and therefore the country, was available. Dropping everything (I doubt she had the luxury of scheduling time to be my host), Mary was at my hotel two hours later and driving me to the hospital. It was only three stories high, but its wide façade went on and on and lent it an immensity that hinted at its importance. It could only hint and no longer proclaim because the façade, clearly once white, stretched out left and right from a main entrance shorn of its doors. We also parked next to a crater in the middle of its lawn, the origins of which I respectfully avoided asking about, but which I assumed was a remnant of the war.

The darkness and pungency of the halls transported me to so many hospitals in so many places I had been while steering us to the medical director's office, where Mary left me in the hands of the medical director's secretary and encouraged me to text her when I was done. When she closed the door behind her, the divide between the humid hall and the air-conditioned office left me feeling like I had been sealed in a walk-in refrigerator. The secretary's engagement in deskwork to the exclusion of small talk added to the chill, and so I busied myself taking in posters about contraception and prenatal care. After someone left the inner office located behind the secretary's desk, a heavyset gentleman in suspenders and a bowtie emerged and silently handed her a paper that she received knowingly, upon which the secretary directed his attention to "the doctor from America." Dr. George Ali begged my patience and left the office suite, returning ten minutes later with two bottles of soda and asking me into his office.

We shook hands after he rounded his desk and put the drinks down.

"Welcome, my friend, to our great country and yes, our great hospital," he proclaimed, throwing up his uplifted arms to each side in a commercial-ready pose.

"Thank you, Dr. Ali. I appreciate your hospitality and for taking the time from your busy schedule on such short notice."

"Ahhh, yes, well, I know your time is precious. So, tell me what has led you to share some of it with us?"

I offered my spiel about my global mental health program and its aspiration to "help make sure everyone, everywhere has access to mental health care."

"And when Mary called, you came! Good man, you are. And oh, that Mental Mary, she needs all the help she can get before she goes mental, you know!" Once his chuckling subsided enough that he was no longer bouncing in his seat, Dr. Ali got down to business and asked, "So, how will talking with me, an obstetrician who runs a general hospital, help you to help her?"

"Well, there's no way mental health professionals alone can tackle the mental health problems here or anywhere in the world, America included, without the help of our fellow health professionals." Dr. Ali looked puzzled, and so, I went on quickly, "The more our colleagues can feel comfortable dealing with mental health issues in their patients without having to rely on mental health professionals, the more people get help."

"Ok, so do you want your baby delivered by a psychiatrist?" Dr. Ali countered, this time without any evident attempt at humor.

"No, I'll take you, if you will," I readily admitted. "But you do use midwives, physician assistants, family medicine doctors to deliver babies. I learned in medical school that one does not have to be an obstetrician to help a woman through a normal, uncomplicated delivery. What I am saying is that for the less complicated psychiatric cases, for issues that may come up in their existing patients, plenty of doctors can help."

"Well, good doctor, I had no psychiatry at all in medical school, but you surely had obstetrics and psychiatry. I have nothing against your psychiatry, but you know that in this part of the world, most of us do not get exposed to it in our training."

"Dr. Ali, you have hit the nail on the head, if you know that phrase." And I am making you nervous... but I suppose I would be, too, if you asked me to deliver my pregnant patients' babies during a psychotherapy session. "That is exactly what my psychiatric colleagues and I strive to do, which is to educate other doctors and health professionals about basic psychiatric diagnosis and treatment. I did not come here to treat patients—that would be a losing battle for little old me. But to share my knowledge...."

Dr. Ali chewed on that and then came alive. "You want to teach us, hmmm? Let me get my staff together." He ambled out of the room, sounded like he was giving some directions to his secretary, and then returned and announced, "The staff will gather in one hour to hear from you." One hour?? About what? I gave voice to the latter question, but Dr. Ali flicked a hand and said, "You are the expert, you tell us what we need to know" as he dismissed me.

I returned to the refrigerator to await my star turn and was not as anxious as you might think. My psychiatric colleagues and I come prepared to give lectures and trainings—these are the stuff of what we do. Usually, we talk through in advance what the educational needs are and prepare materials. Many trips have a theme like addictions or child mental health. But we have learned that we inevitably get surprise requests for topics, although rarely on an hour's notice. Over the years we have accumulated all sorts of lectures on a flash drive for just such scenarios, bringing it with us as regularly as we bring antimalarial medications. And I had said flash drive in my blue-gray duotone knapsack, the same knapsack I have been traveling the world with since I first responded to an earthquake in El Salvador twenty years ago. I keep the knapsack with me at all times since it has my money, passport, and importantly for the moment, my laptop. It also houses my nutrition bars, and I munched on one as I chewed on what I was going to say.

At the appointed hour, Dr. Ali emerged and bade me to follow him. We arrived at a large low-ceilinged room that was neither auditorium nor cafeteria and must have been their all-purpose meeting space. Plastic white chairs were arranged in rows on each half of the room with an aisle through the middle, down which we strode wedding style with me in the rear, groomsman to his groom. Dr. Ali marched with his chin propped up by pride.

The room was packed with about a hundred or so people, and I wondered how the hospital could possibly be functioning without them. It was easy to tell who was who. Nurses were in all-white blouses and skirts, wearing white nurses' caps not seen in the United States for a long while since they were deemed unhygienic. Doctors wore traditional long white coats and serious faces. There were also a few men dressed in everyday clothes. I have no idea how they all gathered so quickly since I heard no overhead announcement, and I was pretty sure they had no idea why they were gathered. But despite that, I was sure I discerned some excitement in the air.

The hospital did have a set-up to project slides on a card table facing a rolled-down screen with a slight tear in the upper left hand, and I popped in my flash drive after saying a prayer to the electronic gods that their computer would not infect it with a virus (I have had a flash drive wiped out on a trip in the Caribbean). Given all the country had been through, I had decided to give a talk on post-traumatic stress disorder (PTSD).

Dr. Ali greeted everyone and introduced the proceedings with such brevity that I felt like a vitamin being forced on a child—who needs explanations when you're going to take it anyway? The "psychiatric specialist from the United States who will now teach us about mental health" began by explaining a little more about who I was and what I was up to running around their country and then I launched into my talk on PTSD.

I tried to make it interactive and started with questions. "Who can say what post-traumatic stress disorder is?" Silence. "OK, why don't we start by defining what a trauma is?" Silence. I quickly realized this audience is surely used to being lectured to and learning in a top-down fashion. Much of the world does not embrace Americans' attachment to being heard. So I launched into what many, myself included, would call "death by PowerPoint." Slide after slide discussing trauma as the experience of a threat to one's life or limb; the healthy "fight-or-flight reaction" to such a threat; how PTSD is a fight-or-flight reaction that does not stop even when the threat does; the four clusters of symptoms that constitute PTSD (intrusive symptoms like nightmares; avoidant symptoms like being afraid to leave one's home; overly negative feelings and thoughts that can look much like clinical depression; and hyperarousal symptoms such as insomnia because someone is too on guard); and the treatment of PTSD with psychotherapy or medication. Just those few sentences alone could put you to sleep.

Throughout, the hospital staff looked back at me without evident emotion, as cool as the air was hot. Yet, only one or two dozed, and no one was checking their cell phone even though they were as prevalent here as they were back home. Most striking was how a good many of them were taking notes on memo pads they had brought along, interrupting their writing only to fan themselves with those pads. The impassive faces of many belied the feverish note-taking occurring just below, like the proverbial duck feet paddling away beneath the placid surface of the water. And I was reminded of something I had seen so many times before in so many desperate places around the globe—an inspiring thirst for learning, any learning, psychiatry, or whatever. That was why Dr. Ali's introduction was so brief—the lecture was no pill being shoved down their throats but rather hydration for parched throats. Whatever it means for ongoing patient care, hospitals like this one grind to a halt at the chance for a lecture, any lecture (as much as I would like to think it were psychiatry they were showing up for).

The inspirational music that was building in the background of my mind paused when about one-third of the attendees opted to leave after I announced the end of my formal talk and encouraged people to stay if they wanted to ask questions. Dr. Ali also looked a bit diminished by the behavior of his minions. But the music picked right up when hands actually started going up. A couple of questions stand out in my memory.

From a doctor: "Sir, what if the person in question is surrounded by traumas that do not stop? How can you call their reaction post-traumatic?"

"Excellent question. It's so important to distinguish normal or adaptive reactions to a trauma from excessive ones. Someone should be on high alert if the threat is ongoing. But we might consider it hyperarousal, as opposed to arousal, if it is not helping them and maybe even if it is harming them. I think of the person who stays up at night watching out their front window for intruders after their home has been broken into rather than leave it to the police and get some sleep." Was that the best example in a place where the police are often understaffed or corrupt?

From a woman in a brown blouse: "You sayin' you can help fear wit talk or pills? You don't need no drinkin'?"

I almost laughed thinking we were sharing a joke, but I managed to catch myself when no one else laughed. Much of the audience looked back at me with inquiring eyes, while several of the white-clad attendees seemed to wince or look down at their laps in dejection. After too long of a pause while I read the mood in the room, I answered the question head-on:

"Thank you for your question. Yes, we can actually treat fear and anxiety. Some fear and anxiety are a normal part of life, and we should be grateful for that since these emotions help us to know when danger or stress is coming our way. But when we get so fearful or so anxious that we can't think straight, can't sleep, can't go about our lives, and then maybe even turn to drinking to help, that's when you should talk to a healthcare professional. There are ways we can talk with you or prescribe medicine to help." Should I have mentioned traditional healers?

I got a nod of gratitude from her, and when we eventually wrapped up, a few people came up and thanked me. As Dr. Ali was escorting me to the main entrance of the hospital where the ever-responsive Mary was going to pick me up, a doctor called after us.

"Excuse me, sir. I am Dr. Robinson. Will you be coming back again?" he asked.

"I certainly hope so," I responded, leaving things open, as I was not sure where he was coming from.

"Well, if I may Dr. Ali," he said nodding to the boss, "It would be an honor if you could come to my general medicine clinic and see patients with me."

Amazing! "Well, Dr. Robinson, it would be my honor. With Dr. Ali's permission, I would be pleased to."

Dr. Ali replied, "Of course. Just don't deliver any babies while you are here!" This time, he found great humor in the possibility, leaving Dr. Robinson a little lost.

"Alas, Dr. Robinson, I am not here for very long. When is your next clinic?"

And so, I had my plan for tomorrow morning in the free flow of things I so cherish on these trips. I felt like I could call off Mary and skip with excitement back to my hotel.

Chapter 10

Convergence

I never did skip back to my hotel. But I did opt to walk to the hospital the next day. I was and still am no fan of being chauffeured around like a deity, even if I knew that driving oneself was not recommended for foreigners for reasons that spanned limited traffic signals, even more, limited street signs, and unlimited chaos. And Mary was too underpaid and overworked as a psychiatrist to add being on call as my driver to her job description, however gracious she was being. It was also an opportunity to let go of the handrails of privilege and psychiatry while I did my work in-country. Psychiatry should only measure its value according to that of the life and lives around it. Symptoms and diagnoses are psychiatrists' lingua franca, but people speak the language of daily life, whose vocabulary includes safety, security, physical health, prosperity, and well-being. All of this influences the health and mental health of people far more than what any health professional of any kind can accomplish. I must admit there's more to life than psychiatry.

As I walk, I cannot help but think that the feverish density of everyone's trying to get somewhere contributes as much to the ever-present heat of the place as the sun above. Some walk slump-shouldered, some with verve. The way trucks and cars forged through the river of humanity would definitely have made me apprehensive to drive—people did not seem to get out of the way until they felt

Unseen: Field Notes of a Global Psychiatrist
Craig L. Katz
Copyright © 2025 Jenny Stanford Publishing Pte. Ltd.
ISBN 978-981-5129-42-7 (Hardcover), 978-1-003-56767-7 (eBook)
www.jennystanford.com

the heat of the automobile engine on them. Adults and children alike peddled their wares, whether sitting off to the sides of the clamor on blankets or fanning it by daring to stop in the middle of it all and approach people of promise like me. I still felt safe opting for a few bananas since, as they say of the developing world—"peel it, boil it, or don't eat it." I needed the energy to avoid the undertow of the crowds.

Walking without the benefit of regular street signage is not much easier than driving except you do not have to worry about distracted driving. But Mary had texted me a combination of street names, counted blocks, and landmarks ("left at the broken lion statue, NOT a right at the intact one") that steered me to the general hospital with precision a pulsating 1 hour later. I needed more help finding the primary care clinic, and when I got there, it looked like my fellow pedestrians beat me here—all of them. It was packed, but I navigated my way to Dr. Robinson and the refuge of his examination room.

That's when I learned Dr. Robinson was expecting me to see patients myself. When he had asked me to come see patients with him, he meant concurrent with his seeing patients. I explained to him that we do not typically get involved in direct patient care given our limited resources and time and only see patients in so far as a local practitioner can apprentice with us. Dr. Robinson half-chuckled, "If only, my good friend!" and elaborated how neither Dr. Ali nor the waiting room full of patients would truck his taking time to learn in the clinic. When I followed with a question about how he was going to figure out which patients I was going to see given this was a primary care clinic, not a mental health clinic, it seemed his enthusiasm for our collaboration had outstripped his planning and provided me with a covert teaching moment.

I suggested we hand out depression surveys in the waiting room for patients to complete while they wait to see Dr. Robinson. Despite my lecture, I did not think we should start by screening for PTSD but rather much more prevalent depression. I could teach the nurses to score them, and they could refer me to anyone who met the threshold for possible clinical depression. If I was able to confirm what the piece of paper suggested, then I would discuss with Dr. Robinson the treatment options. Dr. Robinson loved this, and I felt good that I was going to help the hospital pilot screening for depression in their primary care clinic, something that is endorsed by the World Health Organization.

The good news was that I had brought along a depression survey known as the Patient Health Questionnaire that had been tested across many cultures and translated into many languages with success. The bad news was that it was on my flash drive—I was caught with no paper copies. Dr. Robinson assured me Dr. Ali's secretary could print some for me, and off I dashed, already beginning to find my way around. My excitement skidded to a halt when his secretary informed me the printer was reserved for "executive administrative matters." With Dr. Ali nowhere in sight, I was able to get her to agree to print one page for me and then eek out intelligence about a grocery store across from the hospital that was reputed to have a functioning photocopier. Fueled by my mission, I nearly leapt over the crater in the front yard and found the store, where the rumors were true. The shopkeeper made forty copies for me on a tabletop machine beneath a handwritten sign hanging from the ceiling that declared, "Photographic copies" and pointed downward.

When I got back to the clinic, the waiting room was living up to its name, as it seemed everyone was still waiting. The nurses did not seem troubled by this and sat with me as I reviewed the plan for distributing, collecting, and scoring the surveys. The Patient Health Questionnaire-9, aka the PHQ-9, consists of nine questions representing the nine possible symptoms of Major Depression, the official name for the most common form of clinical depression, and patients are asked to indicate the frequency with which they experience each over the last two weeks. The options are "not at all", "several days", "more than half the days", "nearly every day", which are scored as 0, 1, 2, or 3, respectively. Add up the nine individual items, and if someone scores 5–9, they may have mild depression and 10–14, moderate depression, while scores of 15 or more begin to reflect the likelihood of a more severe condition. Anyone with a total score of 5 or more or who indicates anything other than "not at all" on the ninth question, about suicide, should have been sent my way.

I went to the office set aside for me and prepared for the onslaught I was sure would happen the moment you begin to ask about such a globally prevalent condition in a country that is more or less a mental health blank canvass. Depression is one of the most common causes of distress and dysfunction in the world. Yet, I sat and sat, starting to feel a little depressed myself. Finally, a nurse brought a patient in.

A heavyset woman who appeared to be on the other side of middle age propelled herself in with a cane and dropped into a seat, asking, "Doctor, I no understand what dis? Why dey give it to me?"

Miss Odeh could not read, and when she asked a nurse to decipher the paper that had dropped into her lap, it appears the nurse just whisked her to me without explaining. When I told her it was a survey to find out how she was feeling emotionally, she responded with a "Hmmm" and then demanded, "Why can't dey go on and just go ask me?" Great question!

I told this adorable sage this was the very question I have been spending my career trying to answer. Then I gave one answer—that there are just not enough doctors.

"We're here now ain't we?" Ms. Odeh was not asking to sign up for my public health class, Introduction to Global Mental Health.

And so, I read each question from the PHQ-9 to Ms. Odeh, reminding her of the four possible answers after each of the first few questions until she no longer responded to this forced choice with an "Hmmph" and began to answer on her own. Her score was a 3, and I told her she seemed to be in better mental health than me but asked what she thought about this. She squinted at me, declared "Now, I gotta get dis knee checked out," and made her way back to the waiting room as quickly as that knee would allow.

That line to see me still had not formed, and I decided to investigate. That's when I learned from the nurses that most people did not have a pen or pencil with which to complete the survey. For some reason, the nurses had not felt the need to alert me, nor had they appeared to have given even much thought to trying to remedy the matter. Maybe I should have lectured on depression the day before rather than going with the sexier topic of trauma. After I got past the impulse to go complain to Dr. Robinson and the subsequent more sympathetic thought that maybe the nurses should themselves be completing the PHQ-9, I asked if they could locate some writing utensils. I had a pen in my knapsack but did not feel it fit for sharing as it had remnants of gum stuck to it from trips past. The nurses came up with one blunt but functional pencil and a ballpoint pen imprinted with "Bank of North America" whose journey here must have been an interesting story.

I went out to the waiting room and proudly announced the availability of the pen and pencil but got no reaction. Ms. Odeh chided her peers, "You all let dis doctor help yah. Dat piece of paper it done tell you how you feel in yo heart." Given what I had seen so far of the operations here, it dawned on me that the nurses could well have distributed the survey without even explaining its purpose. I riffed on Ms. Odeh:

"You all have no doubt come here because something is hurting you or giving you trouble. Well, this paper we gave you is about a different kind of trouble, a trouble in your heart that's about feeling sadness that won't go away, about when you can't get life's troubles out of your mind. There's help for this kind of problem, but first we got to know you're having the problem. If you fill out the survey, it can tell us.... So, who wants a pen or pencil to fill it out?" I gave the pencil and pen to two of the five hands that went up out of the forty or so patients and asked them to share. I also told them to hand their completed survey to the nurses.

I eventually got back three surveys—two only had names on them and one had a name and two of the nine questions filled out. As self-doubt coursed through my veins to the point of hypertension, a gentleman knocked on the door. He doffed his baseball cap and introduced himself as "Sam Ervil Gaye." Sam wanted to know if I could help him fill out the survey. Oh, I sure can!

Mr. Gaye sat down, and we went through it question by question with ease, as he obediently accommodated to the format. When we were done, his answers tallied up to a concerning 17 (moderately severe depression). He endorsed problems with having little interest or pleasure in doing things, trouble concentrating, having little energy, poor appetite as "nearly every day" (3+3+3+3=12), feeling down and having trouble falling asleep "more than half the days" (2+2=4), and thinking he would be better off dead for several days (1).

I looked up and asked, "Sam, do you think you need help with your heart?"

"Don't know sir, but yeah…. Here, doctor, I done got dese last time from Dr. Ahmed but dey no help. He say I no have malaria. I come back now. What you think?" Sam implored as he handed me a bottle labelled "ferrous sulfate."

"Well, Sam, it looks like you got these two weeks ago, and it may be too soon to see if they're going to work. But did the doctor check your blood?"

"Yes, sir. Den he done give me dat."

I went through the symptoms Sam endorsed one by one to confirm Sam's experience with each, since the survey only suggests the presence of symptoms and diagnoses that then need confirmation by a (trained) human being. It sounded like fatigue (even more than he would have expected given his sleep problems) and loss of interest troubled him most. As for the suicidality, Sam admitted he even sometimes had thought about taking his life with his scythe but that this never felt like a serious thought. He recounted his separation from his family and how he lived to be reunited with his wife and kids. Although the survey focused on the last two weeks, according to the minimal duration for having clinical depression, it sounded like his symptoms went back months, since the separation.

Ideally, I would have reviewed Sam's medical chart to ascertain what potential medical causes of Sam's symptoms had been evaluated, which is psychiatry 101, but finding that needle in the haystack of the hospital could have consumed the rest of my time in-country. It sounded like the doctor had only evaluated him for malaria and short of that, had given him iron pills in the name of just doing something—I had seen this before. Anyway, if Sam were anemic and if it were due to iron deficiency (the most common cause), it would take 3 months for the iron to actually make a difference, whereas he had been given 24 pills. Back home, I would have been sure to check basic labs such as blood count, blood sugar, and thyroid function, since abnormalities in any can make someone feel depressed. But nothing in his history suggested these were likely, and the scope of his symptoms and the stress of being separated from his family all hung together in a convincing enough picture of Major Depression.

I announced my diagnosis to Sam: "Sam, I also think you need help with your heart. You are experiencing something we call Major Depression. Like I said earlier out in the waiting room, this is where a sad situation feels sadder than it has to feel. Of course, you miss your family. But when you miss them so badly that you lose your will for doing things and feel it in your body, it's gone too far. None of that's going to help you bring your family back. What do you think, Sam?"

"The good Lord, he know you wise," Sam allowed. "What da help?"

I explained medicines can help but knowing that it was not an option here, elected not to discuss psychotherapy since that just felt like a tease. I excused myself to go discuss the medication options with Dr. Robinson, per plan, but he had no idea. I could not tell if that was from a lack of training or experience, but he was too busy for me to get into it. He referred me to the pharmacy and offered up a nurse to escort me there. I first detoured to apologize to Sam for keeping him waiting, but that seemed to confuse him.

George the pharmacist greeted me with enthusiasm, one light bulb that still shone brightly in a place where so many others had burnt out. When I explained who I was and that I wanted to know what the antidepressant options were, I thought he was going to salute me as he turned on his heels to face his wares and call them into action. He came back with the excitement of a dog having retrieved a bone, plopped a single bottle on the counter, and announced, "amitriptyline at your service!"

I should have known not to expect options and was unsurprised that this was it, an antidepressant that is so sedating and laden with side effects at higher doses that back home in psychiatry we mostly just use it for helping patients sleep. It's also a member of a class of antidepressants known as tricyclics, distinguished by the need to check blood levels, an option that was surely not available there. Nonetheless, the World Health Organization has for many years included amitriptyline on their Essential Medication List that guides Ministries of Health around the world, and it is one of the psychotropic medications among the already skimpy menu of WHO's psychotropic recommendations that is fairly consistently available wherever I travel. WHO also features amitriptyline as one of two possible antidepressants in guidelines it publishes for helping non-mental health professionals seeking to treat depression. The chasm that lies between WHO mental health guidelines, to the extent that they are followed around the world, and practice in the U.S. often leaves me calling it the Rest of the World Health Organization, a moniker that sometimes may be to the detriment of the world and sometimes to the exceptionalist U.S.

I looped back to the clinic and asked Dr. Robinson to fill out a prescription (I had not applied for a temporary medical license and hence lacked prescribing privileges) and brought that and Sam back to George.

"Sam, this medicine should help you feel better," I assured him, as we all stood around the pharmacy counter. "You will take a single 25 mg capsule and increase by another 25 mg capsule every few days or so as tolerated up to 100 mg. It won't work right away but we could know in 1-2 weeks if it's beginning to work. But it could take as long as a month of taking it every day to know for sure. And you will know it's working if your heart begins to feel better and you start to get your energy back. On the other hand, it can bother you at first, causing problems like dry mouth, constipation, or too much sleepiness. But if we're lucky, it will sedate you just enough to help you sleep better."

I then asked Sam to do what we call a "teach back" and tell me in his own words how he would be taking the amitriptyline. When he answered, "Just how you do say, doctor," I simplified it and said he should take one pill at bedtime for five days and increase by a pill every five days up to four pills. He was able to teach that back to me. But just in case, I asked Sam to take down my in-country cell phone number and text me if had any questions. This was a courtesy not always extended to "clinic patients" even back in the U.S., where they had to traverse an obstacle course of phone trees and staff to try to reach their psychiatrist. But I refused to offer two-tiered care here, there, or anywhere.

Grateful, Sam left, and I thanked George, who told me he had jotted down my phone number in hopes we could stay in touch. Back in the clinic, I dutifully wrote a quick note for Sam's chart and after snapping a photo of it on my smartphone, took a leap of faith in turning it over to the nurses for putative incorporation into his wayward chart. Now I faced a decision—whether to keep pitching the depression screening protocol to the staff and patients or call it a day? The waiting room had miraculously emptied itself down to about 20% of its capacity, but so had my gas tank. I decided to fold my cards and walk away with gratitude for an invaluable learning experience and a chance to help a lost soul find himself.

But I admit that this time after I said goodbye to Dr. Robinson, there was definitely no skipping back to my hotel.

Chapter 11

Orphanage

With a number of activities under my belt—visiting the psychiatry hospital, observing the mobile psychiatry outreach, lecturing at the general hospital, and trying to launch depression screening in the general medical clinic—I was still feeling like a tourist. I had not yet found a foothold where I thought my program and I could make a long term difference. In Wheel-speak, where was the human resource my program and I could reasonably educate, inspire, and nurture over time and visits in order to make a decent dent in the mental health gap? It was time to check in with Mary. We had only gotten up to discussing Mr. Gibson's allegations of mistreatment at the psychiatric hospital when George the pharmacist called. My immediate thought was that he wanted to form an association of the eager whose founding members were George, Mary, and myself. Instead, he wanted to talk about his brother, a former child soldier now living in an orphanage out in the bush. He was pretty sure he needed a psychiatrist; would I mind evaluating him?

Dr. Robinson, George, and Sam all demonstrated something I have long observed about psychiatry. No matter how unrecognized, underfunded, and misunderstood psychiatry was in just about every place I have been, in the U.S. and abroad, if you show up, they will

Unseen: Field Notes of a Global Psychiatrist
Craig L. Katz
Copyright © 2025 Jenny Stanford Publishing Pte. Ltd.
ISBN 978-981-5129-42-7 (Hardcover), 978-1-003-56767-7 (eBook)
www.jennystanford.com

show up. Hang up a shingle, and they will knock on your door just like Sam did. And the flexibility we build into these trips to be able to take on requests like George's not only affords us completely unforeseen opportunities to learn about mental health in far-flung places but also are a welcomed change of pace for someone like me, whose days back home are scheduled to the half hour with either patients or meetings for weeks to come. Of course, some might say that I am not keeping my eye on the prize of systemic change in chasing after requests like George's that don't promise any clear systematic yield beyond helping one soul. And I myself wonder if sometimes I enjoy the flexibility of these needs assessment trips more than I should.

So it was that the next day George picked me up in a car he borrowed from a friend. Other than my trip in from the airport, I had more or less traveled along two very insular axes within the capital so far—hotel to psychiatric hospital and hotel to general hospital (my day with the mobile outreach team was mostly a rural outing). However adventurous I had been in walking to and from the general hospital, I was now clearly outside of the bubble and my comfort zone as we chugged through streets lined with piles of rubbish that ran on so long and so high it almost gave the impression of mountains of snow formed from post-blizzard street plowing. Of course, that was no snow, and if anything, it seemed like the sun had cooked the rubbish into a banquet that the many goats could nibble on as they strolled without a care in the world. I myself had a lot of cares, especially how our air-conditioner-less conveyance felt more like an earnest amalgam of some of that trash than a steed made of automobile parts. If not for our speed, we could easily have been mistaken for part of the streetscape.

We eventually cleared the city limits and reached a one-lane highway, and the three-hour drive that followed gave George plenty of time to fill me in on how his brother, Amadu, got caught up in their civil war as a combatant. As members of the wealthy minority, Buzzards were able to recruit kids like the nine-year-old Amadu with promises of a better life beyond the oil and rice fields that their parents labored in if they would join them and fight against the Bustards. Before they handed the kids guns and machetes, these men gave them a taste of the wealth to come with surreal parties where it was hard to tell if the thumping was the blaring bass of the music or gunfire from nearby fighting. That taste included drugs, and when the kids quickly became hooked, if the allure of future wealth did not motivate them to enjoin the battle, the immediate need to feed their addiction did. Families and the social fabric were fractured and—worst—child soldiers were literally fighting their parents.

When Amadu showed up back at their parents' home after the war, he was both taller and lesser. Unsure whether to empathize with or seethe at Amadu, their parents reluctantly took him back in for what proved to be a short-lived reunion. Amadu was alternately withdrawn and raging, and the only sense his parents could make of his transformation was that he had been possessed. This also helped them rationalize his involvement in the war in the first place—spirits had gotten hold of him. But the rationalizations lost their traction when a local faith healer's ministrations were unable to exorcise Amadu of his demons. At this point, more frightened for what might happen than sad for what did happen, Amadu's parents asked him to leave.

As the eldest brother, George took Amadu in. But their fraternity wilted in the face of two issues. First, George was no more able to manage Amadu than were his parents. Amadu refused to go back to his recently re-opened school. George had no idea how Amadu spent the day when he was at work and coming home one day to find the ashen remnants of a blanket that he had set afire did nothing to fill in the blanks except with fear. Second, George was defying his parents, and they very quickly figured out his secret. George turned to their priest, who said he knew of a fellow clergyman who was rehabilitating child soldiers out in the country. We were on our way to visit Amadu in the very same car in which George had dropped him off some six months ago.

I have relayed George's account of Amadu without the interruptions George encountered in the telling of it as we drove. Things had certainly sped up when we hit the open highway, but it came in fits and starts as we encountered checkpoints along the way. At the first stop, I was surprised the officials were not wearing uniforms and then apprehensive when they asked George to step out of the car. There was a lot of chatter and a fair amount of finger-pointing back at the car. Then, one of the officers came over to the car, bent over, and looked me over without saying a word, like they were trying to figure out the species of a fish in a low-set home aquarium. I was not sure whether to look ahead or back and opted for a flirtatiously half-hearted wave and quick eye contact. After we drove through in an uneasy silence and were a few miles out, George cursed, "Asshole gangs."

We must have repeated this routine four or five times, and I confess that to my eyes the gang members had a certain uniformity to them even without formal uniforms. String-bean thin and usually clad in white tank top t-shirts, semi-automatic rifles dangled around their shoulders as did cigarettes from their mouths. They were keeping an eye out for rival gangs, and worse, undercover soldiers seeking to infiltrate their territory. And it appeared that being a white guy was too good of a disguise to be true and provided us with comparative ease in passing muster. I was our very own EZ-Pass!

I guess George must have explained to them where we were headed because no sooner had we finally gotten off the highway that we were pulled over once more, and this time they asked me to step out of the car. I did not feel fear but instead tremendous guilt for having put myself in harm's way with my kids and wife back home, having long supported my wandering and always providing a welcome home befitting a hero. The two men actually did not introduce themselves, and even though they wore short-sleeved button-down shirts and slacks and looked more like young computer technicians, I assumed they were gang members of a higher order who decided to vet the reports about us from their underlings. They even had three roadside lawn chairs readied for the chat.

"What brings you to our neighborhood?" one of them began without ceremony and with what I thought was either a hint of skepticism or my operating under the influence of watching one too many television interrogations.

"I am a psychiatrist from America here to help in any way I can. George has asked me to come evaluate his brother who's been staying at the local church," I responded oh so earnestly.

"How do you know Father Reginald?" he went on.

"I don't, but I am looking forward to meeting him. It sounds like he's truly doing God's work," I answered with the hope that flattery, which I admit was heartfelt, would play well.

"He is, he is. May I see your cell phone… unlocked?"

I passed him my cell phone, wishing he had not missed the chance to see the photo of my family that graced the locked phone's screen. He thumbed through a few screens and then passed it back to me.

Then his partner asked, "I heard that psychiatrists could read minds. Can you read mine?"

I tried not to smile at his innocence and confessed, "I wish I could read minds. None of us can. We count on our patients to share what's going on inside. It's a real partnership."

With that George and I were on our way and arrived at what proved to be a compound just minutes later. An imposing security guard allowed us through the gates, where Father Reginald came out to greet us as we parked on a field of dried-out grass. "Hello George, welcome back. And Doctor, it is very good to meet you. I am Father Reginald. Welcome to our humble sanctuary."

After a bathroom stop and some light chatter over tea and crackers, we began our tour. The compound was rung by cinder block walls topped by broken glass and at its center, the crown jewel, was the church. Around the rear perimeter of the grounds were two buildings that were once the nunneries for sisters who served the local parish. Instead of housing ten nuns each, they now housed thirty children each, about four to a room in what looked like a rather well-improvised arrangement. The few remaining sisters who had not been lost during the epidemic, war, or typhoon lived in the other rooms and supervised the children as best they could. They were assisted by local townspeople who were hired as "mothers" and "fathers" to staff the residences and grounds in twelve-hour shifts. The generous pay provided by church authorities overcame any fears they had of these former child soldiers. Along the front perimeter of the church was a schoolhouse that used to serve only as a place for religious instruction but now also served as the school, to the extent they could get the kids to attend and local teachers to come, and the dining hall. There was a local pediatrician who visited for a weekly clinic. There was definitely no mental health provider here or anywhere.

Each of the kids, now ranging in age from 9 to 17, had come to the Father through a unique route, although the first was not part of any grand plan. A priestly favor then turned into a trickle of referrals, and then a torrent limited not by the big heart of Father Reginald but by the dormitory space. As we wandered around, kids were lying in bed, running around playing soccer of whatnot, or having a snack in the school/dining hall. A few of them approached us and asked who we were. When George said he was Amadu's brother, they went running off to no doubt share this intelligence with Amadu. As did the compound, the kids seemed at least superficially in good order—dressed well, appearing physically healthy, and mostly doing things kids do.

Amadu, however, did not do something kids would do when they had visitors—come running to find us. Maybe it was because this was not exactly visiting day at summer camp, but my psychiatric antenna was up and told me were off to an inauspicious start. Father Reginald therefore ended the tour at Amadu's bed, where we found a glistening mango pit but no Amadu. The Father did not skip a beat, beckoning us to follow him to the church and one of the confessional booths, whereupon he knocked on its door frame of the otherwise curtained off priest's compartment and queried, "Amadu?" The only response were some shuffling noises and a ripple that ran through the curtain.

"Amadu, it's Father Reggie and some visitors. Your brother, George, is here." The ongoing silence forced me to face the pathos underlying the sanctuary's initial waft of serenity.

"Brother, it is George. Long time, no see. I have missed you," George stepped in. After another beat of silence, George tried to draw the curtain. However, like the action–reaction they teach you in physics, a small hand reached around and pulled it back almost instantly. Of course, this was more than physics—it was a reflex Amadu surely had acquired to ensure his psychological safety. It was hard to bear witness to the pain on either side of the curtain, and I motioned to George to introduce me.

"Amadu, I brought a friend. He's a doctor from America. He's come all this way to meet you."

"Go away." Progress!

"Hi Amadu, would you be able to come out so I can meet you?"

"No danks."

I suddenly had the idea to step into the penitent's compartment, which, never having been to one before let alone spent much time in a church, was like crossing into a foreign land within a foreign land. There was no seat, and then I remembered from the movies that one kneels on a step, which felt more natural under the circumstances than standing like I was in a telephone booth.

"Amadu, may I confess something to you?" I kneeled and asked, half-distracted as my mind raced to-and-fro trying to figure out whether inspiration or desperation had taken hold of me.

"What dat?"

"Well, I am a psychiatrist, do you know what that is?"

"No."

"It's a doctor that helps people with their feelings."

"Okay, so what you got to confess?" Amadu said in trying to keep to the agenda.

"I confess I am worried about you," I paused but then decided not to leave it there. "I know you been through a lot—becoming a Buzzard…."

"I ain't no Buzzard!" Amadu's scream echoed through the sanctuary and in the chambers of my heart. Fool for stepping on such a foreseeable landmine!

I paused to let things settle and then apologized, saying "I am sorry, Amadu. But you know, that's just it. I confess I am trying to understand what you have been through, but I cannot do it without you. Without your help, I am helpless."

"How can I help? You da doctor." Then he caught himself and added, "I ain't need help."

"Amadu, how are you feeling?"

"Cool."

"Do things ever feel not cool?"

"Go away, man. Danks."

Something told me words had gotten us as far as we were going to get for today, and I decided to resort to some of the tools of the trade of child psychiatrists—a magic marker and paper. I brought these with me in anticipation of needing to do with 13-year-old Amadu what you might otherwise do with younger kids to help them express themselves. I assumed, given what he had been through, his development had been in many ways arrested at a much younger age precisely because he was being asked to act like an adult and a murderous one at that. I also knew that drawing materials were more of a luxury than a staple.

"Amadu, I am going to leave you with a pad of paper and a pen, because I am hoping you like to draw. They're a gift and you can draw whatever you like. But try to also draw some pictures about yourself and share them with Father Reggie. He will send them to me because I would like to see them." With that I stood up, stepped out, and slipped them under his curtain.

We all went back to Father Reggie's office and debriefed. I could see that George was dejected, hoping I could accomplish far more with Amadu. And to some extent that was my fault—in my desire to help and maybe even play hero, I failed to expectation-set from the outset. I tried to correct my oversight, explaining that psychiatry is not surgery and inevitably requires time and perseverance. I assured George that this was a very good start, and this seemed to hearten him until he asked when I could come back next.

"George, I am not sure I can come back on this trip, as much as I would like to. But I do have an idea," I began. That's when I suggested an idea I had hatched in the course of the touring around the compound as a psychiatric light bulb lit up in my mind. "Father, there's plenty of evidence that you can train non-health professionals to provide psychotherapy. I admit there's far less evidence of doing so with kids, but we do have experience with this in other countries. If I can somehow find the resources to send my team back here in the future to train the sisters and the mothers and fathers in basic child mental health, what do you think?" If I can somehow find the resources to back up my ideas.

"Good doctor, may the Lord bless and protect you and give you the strength to come back and do as you say," Father Reggie responded. And with that, I added an item to my post-trip to-do list.

The next day I received a text message from Father Reggie with a photo of a drawing. It showed a tall stick figure pointing a gun at the head of a much smaller figure.

Chapter 12

Connections

"Hi, it's me again, Molly from Power Up… Powerrrrr Up!" Molly chimed as Sam opened his front door. "I'm here to shine my light on you and see how it's going."

"Hello, mam. How are you?" Sam responded, with a slight bow of the head. What do I tell her?

Sam was nervous. He was not taking his medication. Thankfully, he had not lost his flashlight again. Thinking fast, he asked her to wait and quickly proffered his "torch" and indeed held it upright like a one. "It work good!"

"Great, Sam… great. But how are you working?" Molly went on, staying on task.

"I'm good. Danks."

The silence puzzled Molly and further unnerved Sam. Molly correctly concluded she needed to be more direct, even if she thought they were just having a communication problem.

"So, how did it go at the hospital?"

"The doctor, he was good. Danks for dat."

"What did they do for you?"

"They done check my blood."

"And what did they find?"

Unseen: Field Notes of a Global Psychiatrist
Craig L. Katz
Copyright © 2025 Jenny Stanford Publishing Pte. Ltd.
ISBN 978-981-5129-42-7 (Hardcover), 978-1-003-56767-7 (eBook)
www.jennystanford.com

"Dey gave me a pill to make my blood stronger."

"And?"

"Dey no work. I go back. Doctor from America done give me energy pill."

"What's it called?"

"Dunno, maam."

"Can you show it to me?" I can teach some health literacy!

Health literacy (how much people were able to understand the information necessary to make healthcare decisions) took up an entire day of Molly's training. She loved helping people make healthy decisions. Translating "ivory tower doctor talk" into "plain old people talk" spoke to the community organizer in her. After a few drinks she would also admit to herself that, never being able to get through to her mother about the need to take her psychiatric medications, it was a relief to know that imparting knowledge and resolving misunderstandings could actually make a difference how someone, anyone, followed their doctor's recommendations.

Molly had never heard of amitriptyline, but because Google had, she realized the doctor must have diagnosed Sam with depression.

"Sam, how's it been going with this medication?"

"Honest, Ms. Molly, no good. It stuff me up."

Sam finally confessed he had stopped taking the medication. And health literacy was not the issue. Sam was able to tell Molly exactly what the bottle said to do—how he was supposed to increase the number of pills slowly up to four per day and even recalled how it could take weeks to see if it was really going to work. Sam never got past one pill or a week.

"Sam, so what do you mean it stuffed you up?" Molly asked as she had lots of personal experience asking about side effects but had never heard this one.

"It slow me down—can't dink good. I done think maybe dat would get better—the American doctor said so. But it done slow my body...."

Sam saw the confusion tug Mollie's lips to the left and tilt her head along with them and dutifully went on even while embarrassment weighed down his gaze. "Miss, I couldn't go... I couldn't go bathroom."

"Ah... you were constipated?" she blurted out, this time leaving Sam to mirror her confusion on his face. Molly immediately regretted forcing this confession out of him and then further humiliating him with the self-satisfied glee of her own understanding and a diagnosis clearly beyond his.

Molly's embarrassment for Sam gave way to sadness as he elaborated on how scary this was since the American doctor had not told him that this was a side effect. He had once heard the devil could take hold of your innards. To Sam's credit, he did not just stop the amitriptyline but worked up the courage to return to Londo to admit his infidelity and seek his counsel. Londo surprised him by not only not chiding him but instead empathizing with his seeking out a "doctor of science." After tying a thread around the wrist of Sam's dominant hand and chanting an incantation, Londo put a bow around the entire situation by telling him to stop the medicine.

Enter anger as Molly suddenly fumed, "The healer told you that?!"

"...Ah, yes, mam, he done do dat," Sam replied tentatively, wondering if seeking out Londo was one mistake too many to ask of Molly's mercy.

"Take me to Londo," Molly commanded.

Much of the world relies on traditional healers for all manner of ills, from faith healers to herbalists. They have been practicing for millennia, well before Western "doctors of science" entered the scene. In many places around the world, healers are far more available by orders of magnitude and by dint of their location. They can be readily found in the "bush," whereas physicians are not, instead clustering in major cities.

Londo aptly referenced doctors of science, as Western medical practice eventually evolved into being scientifically based or what is otherwise known as "evidence-based medicine." Traditional healers operate on belief and experience, whereas modern medicine more often than not prides itself on having evolved enough to relegate these to secondary status and sometimes even pretends they do not matter. But my own clinical experience sometimes guides how I care for my patients better than and even in complete contradiction of expert-derived treatment guidelines. My encounters with traditional healers have filled me with disdain (for example, when a boy's screams turned out to be a healer's setting a broken bone in their front yard) and inspiration (standing in a rice field as a faith healer paused from their day job to explain to me the power of faith). But I have held medical colleagues in no less disparate regard.

While it's all too easy to sneer at the therapeutic benefits of breaking a pot of clay or being fanned with peacock feathers, these techniques must do and mean something as they have been around for millennia compared to my upstart field of psychiatry's few centuries. There are even scores of plant-based drugs approved for medical use that hail from folk-medicine practice (although I as yet know of none approved for psychiatric use in particular, although psychedelics like psilocybin seem to be on their way). Mostly, while I think traditional healers could probably use a bit more science, I think Western medicine needs to venerate faith and wisdom no less than it does science.

We have begun to research the overlap between traditional healing and psychiatry, and one healer put it pretty well when we asked them what they would recommend for a case we presented to them of a clinically depressed woman: "She should read good books. She should take medicine. She should also pray."

I look forward to when we can put what we learn about the mental health benefits of traditional healing into practice that benefits the art and science of healing. Healing encompasses any practice that reduces suffering from wounds visible and invisible, even if it was not borne out of a test tube or a clinical trial.

In the meanwhile, the transformed Molly stormed off to Londo like a parent on the trail of a schoolyard bully. If she knew where to find Londo, it would have been easy to imagine her dragging Sam by the hand. Among other things, she was propelled by the premise that traditional healers are as dismissive of physicians as they are of healers, taking Londo's intervention to be narrow-minded interference in Western do-gooding. She had heard stories about healers mucking up the good deeds of NGOs but admittedly never witnessed this herself. Now was finally her chance to right this wrong.

Londo was not at home, i.e., in office. Worn out and scared, Sam hoped this would be the end of it. But a good Samaritan in the house nearby shouted out, "Hey dere Sam. You know Londo not home in de day. He out in dem fields." They pointed "dat way" toward a road leading out of town past the rusted chassis of a car. Sam gave Molly a "well-I-guess-we-will-have-to-come-back-another-day" shrug which she trumped with a "we're-not-done-look," and the forced march resumed.

Sam more or less knew where the fields of interest were, but he had to periodically stop and ask a local resident to reassure himself, especially since he had not been feeling clear-headed for a while. And it seemed each time he did that, they acquired a young escort intent on assuring them safe passage. By the time they got to the fields, five children excited to help him help this white woman were in tow, each angling for a chance to hold Molly's hand. She had to work hard to maintain her war footing amid all of the good cheer.

The kids proved to be a boon in not only getting them to a plantain farm where Londo made most of his living but to the very plot of interest that morning. Molly had no flashlights to spare for their effort but gave them each a piece of chewing gum. This only excited them even more, and they scattered in different directions inspired to search for more benefactors like bees in search of pollen. The diversion they provided also disappeared with them, and it was back to business as Sam doffed his cap and approached Londo.

"Londo, your pardon sir, dis here Ms. Molly, she from de torch company," Sam murmured, sure this was not good.

Londo leaned his machete against a half-sawed plantain tree and extended his hand with such an obvious effort at daintiness that it proceeded in slow motion. "Ah, the torch company, nice to meet you, Ms. Molly. I hear you have illuminated our community to the great shame of our equatorial sun."

Was this deference or mockery? Molly had no idea whether to pontificate or duel and momentarily defaulted to a watered-down version of her usual amiability and said, "Nice to meet you and thank you for your kind words, Mr. Londo."

When Londo corrected her that it is just "Londo," Molly decided he was mocking her after all and began to berate him about advising Sam to stop the medicine a doctor prescribed and demanded to know why he did not suggest Sam consult with the doctor.

"Madam Molly, I did suggest that." As Molly recalibrated, Londo went on. He recounted how he asked Sam if had spoken to his doctor and that Sam said the doctor was too far away and that he could not afford to travel to see him again. So, he asked Sam to fetch the bottle of medicine to see if he could make any sense of it. When Sam returned with the bottle and Londo opened it to take a look, he extricated a paper curled around the circumference of the bottle that had the doctor's phone number on it. Sam had tucked it away there but despite this bounty, Sam never tried to call him and even in the face of Londo's urging would still not do so nor even let Londo try.

Molly's mind raced while Sam considered whether to race away. Then the wounded plantain tree snapped, and its fruit-bearing top crashed to the ground, breaking the spell and compelling Sam to amend the record:

"Maam, that doctor did gone and give me his phone number. But maam, you see, I don't never call a doctor in my life."

Molly had lots of practice and no such hesitation. She shifted gears into the fed-up parent who had the principal on speed dial for a hapless student and rang up on the doctor on the spot. I was in my hotel room ahead of an afternoon meeting at the Ministry of Health when the phone rang. Molly introduced herself and breathlessly summarized the journey of my prescription. She agreed to turn on the video on her phone and put on Sam so he could tell me what happened in his own words. I have done plenty of telepsychiatry but never with plantain trees as my patient's backdrop.

"Doctor, sir, I got all stuffed up."

"What do you mean, Sam?"

"I could not go to the bathroom."

"You mean you were constipated?"

"What dat?"

"You could not move your bowels?"

He gave me a quizzical look apparent even on the small screen of my phone.

"You could not make kaka?"

"Yes, dat right. And it scary. You never told me about dat."

"I told you it could cause constipation."

Fool I am! If I could read his confusion through a phone, why didn't I pick it up in person??

"I am sorry, Sam, I did not explain things well enough. This is a common side effect of this medicine."

"Dank you, sir."

"Sam, how about starting it again?"

"Could I get better energy pill that don't stuff?" And don't get de spirits mixed up in it?

"Sam, I don't have other pills right now. We got to make this work."

Sam had no chance to respond, as he disappeared in a kaleidoscope of herky-jerky images and ruffling sounds. When things leveled off, Sam was replaced by a man with a booming voice. I had no idea anyone else had been there and thought I was about to hear a ransom demand.

"Doctor, I am Londo. I am the faith healer Ms. Molly just told you about. Nice to meet you, sir. I am trying to help Sam."

"Nice to meet you, Londo. It looks like we are on the same team." Amazing!

"Good doctor, I know how to cleanse the body. Maybe if I do that, Sam will take your pill?" Londo offered.

And that's how I came to partner with a faith healer for the first time, realizing my long-held hope of doing so by sheer luck. I had no idea what Londo planned to do, but Sam accepted it. He would now re-try the amitriptyline. Londo further signed on to monitor him, and Molly agreed to provide Londo with calling cards to put minutes on his phone. Londo would serve as my eyes and ears and call me with updates. This was a global health masterpiece:

Low-income setting + person in need + psychiatrist + healer + NGO + antidepressant + telephone = another plank laid in the bridge across the mental health gap.

I started to envision the case report I could write. But where would Sam fit into my paean to the possible? My inner realist began scripting a counter-story, a dirge of doubt. These were the concerns that could pluck the nails out of the Sam Gaye bridge: 1. Already having a bothersome side effect at the very lowest dose of antidepressant medication, a dose that was nowhere near that required to have antidepressant effects; 2. Uncertainty about the ability of Londo's ministrations to remedy this and even concern for their safety; 3. Side effects that would surely mount as Sam necessarily increased the dose of the amitriptyline; 4. Worst of all, if Sam could not ultimately tolerate the medication despite his best efforts and our model collaboration, I had no backup, no gears to give. Neither the psychiatric hospital nor the general hospital pharmacy had any other antidepressants.

I began to wonder if I was duping more than treating Sam.

Chapter 13

Peanut Butter and Jelly

Even as my trip was rushing past me, it was surely premature to select a paean or a dirge for my trip's theme song. Mary thankfully picked me up shortly after the call with Sam and my new field team, curbing my temptation to weigh the matter further. I not only needed to keep on trucking but to keep my eyes on the road. It was time for my courtesy call with the Ministry of Health.

Health officials from Ministries of Health never seek out my program's help, and although I cannot say for sure why this is, I can surmise: (1) it would be too embarrassing; (2) they are happy to let clinicians in the trenches like Mary solve their problems for them; (3) they do not have to work in psychiatric hospitals or clinics that are busting at the seams. I tend to believe their willful ignorance of the realities of their country's mental health gap is abetted by situating psychiatric hospitals and clinics out of sight as much as possible.

In truth, working with high levels of any government would be a project unto itself, involving bureaucracies and lawyers on both sides of the collaboration. It is for this reason that our global mental health program has never pursued formal agreements with partner countries unless we have to. I therefore confess we have no memoranda of understanding with any of our many partner countries around the world like Doc Mary's. It is bad enough that

Unseen: Field Notes of a Global Psychiatrist
Craig L. Katz
Copyright © 2025 Jenny Stanford Publishing Pte. Ltd.
ISBN 978-981-5129-42-7 (Hardcover), 978-1-003-56767-7 (eBook)
www.jennystanford.com

every time we send a psychiatry resident overseas (or even outside of the walls of our medical center), regulators that oversee residency training in the U.S. require our partners to sign a document known as a "program letter of agreement," the details of which I will not go into beyond saying negotiating the wording of these and securing the various signatures at home and abroad necessary to execute them often takes up as much energy as planning the substance of trips. PLAs make me want to see a psychiatrist.

Our global partnerships usually work out just fine based on a handshake. But we have also learned that getting buy-in from Ministries of Health not only lends more credibility to our projects but also becomes essential when our liaisons like Mary leave their positions, usually from burnout that we are too late to prevent. Collaborations have needlessly collapsed or foundered because we have not done our diplomatic due diligence and established in-country professional relationships beyond our liaison, especially with their bosses. Hence today's visit to see the chief medical officer of the Ministry of Health, Dr. Toussaint, who was unavailable the day Mary rerouted me to seeing Dr. Ali at the general hospital.

The Ministry of Health building was a remarkably unremarkable looking, a two-story beige box befitting an industrial business park. The interior was cold—both the air and the aura—as though it had been vacuum-sealed to prevent the human mess of the Ministry's hospitals and clinics from seeping up the chain. Again, Mary left me to my own devices, this time while she caught up with people and paperwork while on the premises.

The meeting with Dr. Toussaint perfectly captured something I have come to call "PB&J" as well as any other experience I have had. It happens to be true that I find bringing peanut butter and jelly on global health trips to be the perfect snack when neither mealtimes nor safe food are assured. But here PB&J is an acronym for how a successful global health missioner should interact with a country, colleagues, and information while traveling. Much like chunky peanut butter is loaded with peanuts, this PB&J is loaded with should-nots.

P stands for plunderer, and it references our attitude, as resource-richer collaborators, toward our host country. Some writers in the field of global health have charged global mental health practitioners with "medical imperialism" and global health in general with colonialism. No. We should neither come to plunder nor appear as such, seeking not to take but to give, even if we inevitably receive much back in the form of unique professional experiences and gratification as well as the bow we take each time we return home to our more earthbound colleagues. We should therefore also not comport ourselves as tourists, neither taking nor giving, even if we should spend some time getting to know a country outside of the walls of health care. We are visitors, with all the respectfulness that entails, including the burden our visit places on our hosts (I could have called this VP&J, but it does not have the same ring). Since it is our practice to only go to places where we are invited, it is still better to consider ourselves invited guests. Even though Mary had indeed invited us, concerns about plundering presented themselves from the very outset of our dialogue.

"Good doctor, welcome," he declared, standing up from behind his desk to offer me a handshake sandwich as he took my right hand between his two. "How may I help you?"

It sounded like whatever prep Mary had given Dr. Toussaint needed refreshing, and so, I gave much the same introduction to global mental health and my trip as I did Dr. Ali (see Chapter 9 if you would like to hear it again). But I especially emphasized that I was responding to Mary's invitation.

"What will you be doing?" he inquired, and I thought I spied the hint of an arched eyebrow.

"This is an assessment trip. My focus is on figuring out how to match our mental health resources to your needs," I explained.

"Ah, so you will be doing research?"—now his eyebrow arched for sure. We were not dabbling in opening niceties. I have learned over the years that when working with our global collaborators, "research" is met with either paranoia or indifference. Dr. Toussaint exemplified both, in turn.

"Well, we focus a great deal on training—making existing human resources more comfortable working with people with mental health problems and more knowledgeable and skilled in treating those problems. This avoids trying to solve the mental health gap by hiring more people and ignoring why the gap exists in the first place." Now Dr. Toussaint raised his eyebrows in appreciation. "We have trained, sometimes supervised, primary care doctors, nurses, community health workers, but I admit that we have never studied the long-term impact of what we do. In the face of our own limited resources, my colleagues and I have opted to focus on delivering a service more than on studying it."

"So, I imagine you have come here to our fair country to finally get around to your long-delayed study of your best efforts?" Dr. Toussaint pressed, eyebrows in neutral but voice not.

"No, no. Sure a study would be nice, but I do believe there are already enough studies out there to suggest what we do works. We're trying to turn that research into practice. We're here to help," I countered.

"Well, good to hear. We have had researchers come and pick over our country like some curiosity to be turned round and round and then put back down. They quench their curiosity and fatten their academic portfolios and leave," he spat.

"But once I figure out who we could reasonably help train, I would prefer to do a needs assessment, an analysis of their knowledge and attitudes toward psychiatry to figure out what they know and how they feel about psychiatry. That way our training will be on target for their needs," I cautiously elaborated for fear I may yet be tripping a wire.

Dr. Toussaint instead waived me off with a laugh: "Ahhh... who needs that? I assure you no training you do here will be wasted. I may need to sit in myself!"

I resisted my inner nerd and the voice of my dean and did not protest. I understood that the vast unmet needs here informed this "better-than-nothing attitude" even if I aspired to be much more than that.

The B in PB&J is for buddy. It captures how we relate to our host and others in their healthcare system in the course of our collaboration. Ideally, we become friends in the course of a long-term relationship, but we should not expect to start out as buddies. As many commonalities we have as fellow health care professionals and human beings, our professional training and experiences are often worlds apart—consider how Mary's psychiatry training was entirely on the job while I had the benefit of formal education and training in medical school and then residency. And our personal lives are usually vastly different, given the disparate income levels of our respective countries. There is just too much to learn about one another as professionals and as people. On the other hand, we should not stride in as giants who are above it all and potentially foster our host's need to worship us as idols who can make things all better. We come as colleagues, seeking to collaborate around our common aspiration to make the world a healthier place.

Dr. Toussaint suddenly caught himself and apologetically reversed course and said, "So, we got down to business rather quickly. Where are my manners? Tell me about yourself. You have kids?"

I told him about my wife and my young daughter and son and how much I miss them during my weeks away. He told me his wife and four kids are living in Europe while they attend school there and how much he missed them over the years. My longing for my family felt embarrassingly self-involved given the years-long separation Dr. Toussaint was enduring. We were not starting out as bachelor buddies.

It was refreshing to talk about family before talking about our professional selves. That came next. Dr. Toussaint recognized my medical school: "Ah, that's the place where they do cardiology!" True. And psychiatry.

Dr. Toussaint held my home institution in such high regard that he thought the rich American medical school should have the equipment to spare. And how tempted I was to climb onto that pedestal!

Himself an obstetrician, he wondered if I could help him replace the ultrasound machine for the women's hospital he directed until ascending to his role as CMO?

"I wish I could."

Well, given our world-famous cardiology program, how about an echocardiographic machine?

"I will certainly keep my eyes open for one when I am back home."

Would he be able to visit my hospital as an observer in the Department of Obstetrics and Gynecology ?

"That I can work out."

The J in PB&J is for journalist. Since in global health, our patients are communities or countries that are foreign to us, if we stick to our ethos of going only where we are invited, then we should feel not only obliged but comfortable learning about our patients. We should evaluate their system's psychiatric needs and psychiatric resources and the will to narrow the gap between the two and to work with us in so doing. Not spending time learning about our host would be being guilty of said imperialism. But as we drill in on what they want and compel our colleagues to be honest with themselves as much as us about what they really want, we can come across as investigative journalists rather than humanitarians. As we learn, they feel exposed, curiosity becomes snooping, and expertise turns to condescension. It's a proverbial balancing act.

"So, that needs assessment you're doing, yes... what are your observations so far?" Dr. Toussaint asked, inviting me to jump onto the balance beam.

I extolled Dr. Juma's dedication, which was an excellent place to start since it turned out it had been he who recruited her to work in psychiatry. I gushed over the mobile outreach team. I expressed gratitude for having been invited into the primary care clinic.

"So, we have no work for you after all, doctor?" Dr. Toussaint half-laughed in response to my opening tribute.

And so, I leaned in the other direction. When I mentioned the overcrowding at the psychiatric hospital, Dr. Toussaint admitted he had to find some help for Mary.

Feeling I still had my footing, I launched into what was fresh on my mind since my morning and talked about the shortage of medication.

"Dr. Toussaint, getting Mary some additional staffing would be superb. But without a better supply of medication, I am not sure how much better things can get at the hospital."

"Ah, yes. I am not so familiar with your medications, but I know we have a shortage. Mary won't let me forget," he conceded.

I detailed how I had encountered only three medications so far—haloperidol, amitriptyline, and injectable diazepam—and recounted how this meant they only had one antipsychotic, one antidepressant, and an injectable anti-anxiety medication suitable only for hospital care. They had none of the myriad other medication options within these classes and did not even have an entire class of medication, mood stabilizers for manic-depression and aggression. And what they did have were old, side effect–laden medications that would not be anyone's choice if they could only have one of each.

"Maybe I have not seen a representative example of things, but if this is what you have at your only psychiatric facility and your best general hospital, it does not bode well. I am not sure how you could ever truly address your country's mental health needs on the back of a formulary like this," I preached as I began to lose my footing.

"Doctor. Thank you for this... lecture. I no longer feel so badly for missing your presentation to Dr. Ali's staff, which I heard was indeed not to be missed." Word gets around.

The silence lasted a moment too long for me, and I pressed on, asking Dr. Toussaint how much the Ministry budgets for psychiatric medications each year.

"Doctor, that is folded into our overall medication budget, and so I could not tell you. You know, we have shortages of many medications, not just yours. All of our different medical specialties are like my children, and I have to make sure they each get something," he explained, in turns flabbergasting and embarrassing me but then shoving me to the ground with this—"I hear about how problems with the American mental health system feed your country's enchantment with mass shootings. What are you doing about that?"

"Dr. Toussaint, if I only knew. But I will tell you this, it's a lot more complicated of a story than guns and mental illness," I replied and then, regaining my footing, added, "I am just hoping the story of things here is a lot less complicated."

"You are a dreamer, doctor. But that's not such a bad thing," Dr. Toussaint offered. "I wish I could promise you your rivers of antidepressants. Is there not more to psychiatry than pills—all that counseling you do?"

"Yes, oh yes, there is psychotherapy. Talking therapies can make a big difference," I concurred. "A gentleman I have been consulting on as recently as this morning has clinical depression. There's a good chance that the amitriptyline we prescribed will not work out, and then he's out of luck. If he had access to something like cognitive–behavioral psychotherapy, that would be a perfect option. But when you go around the world, psychotherapists are even rarer than psychotropic medications."

"Cognitive–behavioral psychotherapy... hmmm. Is that CBT? Good doctor, your dreams can come true. There was a team here from America some time ago that started a CBT program. You better ask Doc Mary. Your evaluation is not done."

What?

Chapter 14

A Rose in the Garden

I called Mary after I left Dr. Toussaint's office, and she immediately met me back at her car.

With a more cordiality-deficient immediacy of my own, I buckled in and all but demanded to know, "Mary, you have a CBT program here?"

"No, sir. Good Lord, I would have told you," she responded as she steered the car around several goats lingering in the street as though no one was willing to ask for directions.

I then insisted, "Dr. Toussaint said there was a CBT program started by some Americans a few years ago."

"Yah, yah, I heard about that too back when I started talking with the patients in the Treatment Units during the virus," she recounted. "Someone told me they could help the patients like I was. But if Dr. Toussaint told you they would be the solution to this country's mental health needs, he's fooling himself. I found out they up and left about a year before the virus and never came back. That's like four years ago.

"That man likes to think that Mental Mary is the one and only answer to mental health in the country. I am like his sleeping pill—as long as Mental Mary is on the case, he can put his head down on the pillow and have sweet, guilt-free dreams. And whenever he

Unseen: Field Notes of a Global Psychiatrist
Craig L. Katz
Copyright © 2025 Jenny Stanford Publishing Pte. Ltd.
ISBN 978-981-5129-42-7 (Hardcover), 978-1-003-56767-7 (eBook)
www.jennystanford.com

dares drop that charade, instead of reaching into his pocket to pay for more resources, he lands on the most cost-effective solutions of all—imaginary ones. He once had this idea to deal with our rampant alcoholism by asking bartenders to limit how many drinks they serve. Yeah, that way they pay for his program, not him."

I was taken aback by Mary's bitterness, because, while perfectly understandable, it seemed entirely unlike her. But I did my own Dr. Toussaint and ignored her grievances, going on with my agenda. I asked her if she knew what the program was about.

"All I know is that they trained a bunch of people to provide CBT and gave it out for free. Sounds too good to be true, you know? I guess it's no surprise it could not last. The good Lord is eternity but not all his works can be," she sighed.

I had so far not had a eureka moment where a bridge across the mental health gap in the country came into view. The idea of training the mothers and fathers at Father Reginald's compound was exciting but something about it felt pollyannish—they were likely too busy putting out fires and serving meals to be holding psychotherapy sessions. But this was starting to feel like the on-ramp to an idea to run with. I asked Mary if she knew any of the CBT therapists or patients. She did not but promised to look into it.

And so, it was that the next morning magical mental Mary apprised me of one Rose Solomon. According to Nurse Providence's assistant nurse's husband's cousin's herbalist, Rose was one of the CBT psychotherapists. No one knew her address or phone number, but she usually sold fruit in a part of the capital city known as the Garden District. Johnny the nurse assistant and outreach van driver was dispatched to help me find her.

I had so far failed to follow my own advice and take some time to relax and enjoy the country (no matter how impoverished, every place has something to offer). So, I was looking forward to doing double duty while strolling the gardens *en route* to finding Rose. When Johnny parked the van and we began to walk without any gardens in sight, I assumed we were headed to a place so pristine that you could not drive there. But when I asked Johnny how far the Garden District was, he told me we had arrived. To my eyes, it looked like every other commercial street in the capitol with its rows of merchant booths on either side, riverbanks to the roaring rapids of humanity in which auto, farm animals, and foreigners bobbed.

"So, Johnny, why do they call this the Garden District?"

"It's de oldest part of de city, sir. It's like de Garden of Eden," Johnny explained in all seriousness.

To my eyes, we could easily have been re-tracing my steps to the hospital, but thankfully Johnny could see otherwise. Twice he opted to stop and mention Rose's name, and that was all it took to find ourselves standing above Rose. Finding a Rose in the Garden was a feat that put finding a needle in a haystack to shame.

Rose sat below the hubbub on a stool that could not have been more than a foot high, as her bent legs, anchored by dusty brown sandals, angled up so high they jostled with her arm for airspace. She wore a plain black dress over roundish, plump features and was situated in a back corner of a yellow blanket on which fruits and vegetables were organized in neat mounds. I had an image of a giant goddess watching over her mountainous dominion. There were bananas, mangos, star fruit, papayas, and some sort of melon. Pineapples kept guard in a line on both sides of the blanket.

"Hi, you are Rose, Rose Solomon?" I asked in my "sorry to bother you" voice.

"Dat's me. You want fruit? It's de garden's delight," she responded solicitously.

I stuck to the safe-foreigner playbook and bought yet more bananas and shared them with Johnny.

"Rose, I am a doctor from America, a psychiatrist, and I came to meet you because I understand you were trained in cognitive-behavioral psychotherapy," I explained in between bites of the best banana I had ever had.

"Huh? What dat?... Dat not me. Sorry, sir. But I got de best fruit in de garden. Hey, in de city, too. What you like?" she pitched.

Oy. I wasted my precious time. "Excuse my mistake. But I will take some star fruit; we don't get enough of that back home," I replied with as much enthusiasm as I could muster.

Johnny and I turned to slip back into the river of people and begin our trek back to the car. But I suddenly began noticing the heat and feeling dizzy. I asked if we could stop while I drank some cool water from my thermos and dabbed some on the back of my neck. I had enough spare energy to feel perturbed by how untroubled Johnny seemed. Don't you realize what's at stake here?? Aren't you hot??

That's when Rose's voice broke the spell of my self-pity. "Hey, doc, do you mean de talking?"

The heat lifted as suddenly as it came, and I asked, "I think I do, but can you tell me what you mean?" How shrinky I sound.

"Before dat virus some Mericans came and taught me to heal," Rose began. She might as well have turned on some cosmic air conditioner.

Rose recounted how she learned to "heal with words" from the Americans and how they paid her to heal and even initially paid her when she was in what sounded like a several-week training. She said at first someone was always watching her heal and telling her what to do, and after a while, they let her do it herself. But there was always a "boss lady" around before and after each session, asking Rose's clients questions and typing into her computer.

Although I was now fairly certain we had found the very CBT-trained person I was looking for, I opted for certainty in a place lorded over by uncertainty and asked, "How exactly did you use words to heal?"

"People, dey get stuck. I help 'em go free. Dey dink too much in de head. Dey don't look around dem and see what it is, not what dey dink it is," she explained in as no-nonsense and optimistic of a description of cognitive psychotherapy as I ever heard.

Rose was not done and unwittingly addressed the B in cognitive-behavioral psychotherapy as she continued, "Dey get stuck in what dey do, too. Dey done go in circles, but I do tell 'em to stop chasing de tail like some silly monkey. Why don't dey do dis?"

"Rose, where did you get your clients from?" I wondered. I was especially curious about this since I have long thought that the mental health gap will only really get whittled down when a consumer culture grows up around mental health care and people expect it the way they expect to receive health care or running water.

"De boss lady, she done take care of dat. Some of dem real lucky and see me or one of de utter healers. Yeah, but some of dem get a book," Rose explained.

"Ahh, you mean some of the clients were told to get their help from a book... not you?" I clarified, and she confirmed.

That's when I realized this was a research study, which invited a whole new set of questions, (including how I had not come across this before!).

We were interrupted by a customer, and I quickly stepped aside. Johnny did not have to since he had disappeared somewhere. After Rose handed over two melons and dispensed change from a black bucket with "Diamond Paint Company" printed on it in rainbow colors, I stepped forward again.

"Rose, is it OK if I keep asking you questions?" I asked, hoping she would agree but probably planning to do so anyway. Rose nodded for me to go on, and I next asked what happened to the program.

"Well, dey said they done learned what dey needed and dey left. But dey said dey would come back again. And I just come back here to sell my fruit. But dey no come back. You don't know 'em?"

"No, Rose I don't, but I would sure like to. So, they never came back?" I asked even though I already knew the answer.

"No, sir. Dey don't. I dink dat virus done do dat. But do wish dey do call me. I still have de phone," she lamented.

Rose also still had the books they gave her and when she saw how eager I was to see them, she told me her home was just a few blocks away. If I minded her business, she would run and get them.

It somehow felt wrong to sit on Rose's stool, but it also did not feel like it was good for business for a tall white guy to be standing over the fruit and shorter patrons. So, I plunked down and hoped I did not look as silly as I felt peering over my knees. I was selling no fruit and feeling badly for any interruption in business my talismanic presence posed and secretly bought a few mangoes to give to Johnny.

Rose returned with a training manual that was indeed entitled '*Healing Words*' and whose subtitle read '*A Training Manual of the Global CBT Project*'. I thumbed through and found it was a training manual for treating clinical depression. It was filled with descriptions of classic thinking problems such as "black and white thinking" and "discounting the positive." She also had a manual entitled, *Healing Reading*, which must have been the self-help reading material for the control group in the study. It was filled with such topics as explanations of clinical depression and discussions of healthy habits for mental health.

I suddenly wondered whether Rose could read either of these manuals, let alone read, even though I assumed literacy must have been a requirement for participation in the study. Obnoxiously, I asked Rose to point out to me what part of the *Healing Words* manual she found most helpful, and without pause, she flipped open to the chapter on "Behavioral Activation," which is psych-speak for getting people out of bed and active in their life when depression weighs them down and saps them of their drive and energy.

"Doc, dese people, dey done like to be told what to do," she elaborated.

Rose was on her game. After she served another customer who bought one of everything, I therefore finally got to the punch line— "Rose, would you like to be able to work as a healer with words again?"

"Sir, I done been doing it. People come to me with deir problems— neighbors, friends, even some customers ask to speak to me before buying de fruit. Dere's no boss lady and no pay, but I do it and it done feel good," she countered.

"Wonderful, wonderful," I said because it really was, and then went on, "Rose, if there were a way to work as a healer again for pay, would you do it?"

"Oh, yes, sir. Dat is de good Lord's work. You can pay me?" she asked hopefully.

"I wish I could right now, but I am going to go back to America to find a way," I admitted. "And I promise I will try with all my might to come back with good news, God willing! By the way, do you know any of the other healers who were trained?"

Rose did not and bemoaned how the boss lady who probably did had been murdered. Ouch in so many ways.

I took down Rose's cell phone number and saw my way to giving her my business card and then collected Johnny, who was eating steamed potatoes with utensil-free nimbleness at a nearby booth. Being neither so nimble nor so strong of stomach, I declined to share and gave him his mangoes before we were off.

When I got back to the hotel, I set to do a literature search for Rose's study and found it. Why I was not so successful during my de rigueur pre-trip review of relevant psychiatric literature was beyond me and incredibly frustrating. I could have met Rose and begun to seek out her compatriots early in my trip, not days before it was to end.

The paper was colorlessly titled, "A Lay CBT Program for Treating Depression in a Global Setting." As surmised, they had randomized Rose's countrymen with diagnosed depression into a control group and a CBT group. And it was an incredible success, revealing how the lay psychotherapists outperformed the control group who only received self-help reading and occasional meetings with an American staff person to discuss the book. The requisite discussion of the next steps in their conclusion included a plan to expand the program by having the lay psychotherapists train others to provide the service, hoping for a multiplier effect that would eventually render the Americans superfluous. What a model aspiration for any global health professional! Unfortunately, given the date of the publication, it was now a three-year-old aspiration. Almost as unfortunately, their acknowledgments thanked the Ministry of Health for their collaboration but did not mention Rose and her colleagues. I would like to think they did not even share the article with them due to the untimely death of the "boss lady" who must have been the in-country research coordinator.

But rather than look back, I was looking forward, already concocting a plan to build a mental health program around Rose and colleagues. Locate her compatriots; find an in-country coordinator; recruit some in-person trainers to refresh their CBT skills and then telepsychiatry supervisors back home to help translate classroom skills to real world practice; raise funds to pay everyone we can and tap goodwill for the rest. And then I could say *Voila! Mission accomplished!* I felt a familiar shift in the momentum of my trip, having found what looked to me like the catalytic crossroad where what they can, want, and need to do meets what we can and want to do. I felt as much relief as excitement that Mary and I had not come this far in vain.

Chapter 15

Derapy

Amid the gray cinder block walls and corrugated metal roof, the green chalkboard feels like a stalled paint job. If you calculate in the dirt floor of the classroom, the board feels more like a dubious promise. Students are on summer recess, and the classroom has that profound student-less emptiness. The chairs armed with their side desks may be poised row after row like soldiers in formation, but they're dozing on their feet when Sam, Rose, Londo, and I arrive.

How often do I tell my colleagues before sending them out into the world that we do not go to treat patients even if our professional compass always spins us in their direction? Resist the gravitational pull of the black hole that patient care "there" will surely be in order to truly make a sustainable difference! Teach, mentor, advise, build—but do not treat! Well, even if dutiful doctoring makes for hypocritical preaching, we are foremost here to help Sam and, I pray, in the process learn something bigger for my other patient, this country.

The sheer fact of the call I had gotten from Londo about Sam reassured me that the little system of care I had put in place was working. That the call was about Sam's having been unable to stick with the antidepressant due to the side effects would have been more demoralizing but for its predictability. It also came right after I

Unseen: Field Notes of a Global Psychiatrist
Craig L. Katz
Copyright © 2025 Jenny Stanford Publishing Pte. Ltd.
ISBN 978-981-5129-42-7 (Hardcover), 978-1-003-56767-7 (eBook)
www.jennystanford.com

met Rose and was dreaming big dreams, into which Sam's plight got incorporated so quickly it felt more like an opportunity. Wait, I can have Rose treat Sam! Programs have to start somewhere.

And here we are in Sam's town. To get here I bought two days' worth of fruit from Rose to compensate her for the time and then shared it with the patients at the psychiatric hospital. In "exchange," Mary again dispatched Johnny-the-available to drive us. And Londo secured the dormant local school for us to not only meet but sleep— we would be staying over. It was just too long of a drive to do it all in one day. And anyway, Londo asked me to see someone else while I was here who had apparently just been released from Mary's care at the psychiatric hospital. Tomorrow morning.

The others enter the classroom but then look lost, especially Londo who seems as though his visions for the day had just never gone past getting us into the school. I am not sure he understands what we're going to do, and in a sense, neither do I—I only know what I hope we're going to do. I step forward and recruit four chairs for us to sit in a circle. I had already introduced everybody to everybody And so, we get started.

I open: "Sam, do you know why we're here?"

"Dunno, doctor. Sorry I stopped de medicine. I can start again?" Sam confesses.

I pursue: "Sam, why would you want to keep taking something that bothers you?"

"Dunno doctor. Cause you done say so," he offers.

I press on: "Sam, why would I want you to take something that bothers you? Why would anyone?"

"I done wrong. I sorry," Sam confesses.

Instead of crying, I offer an attempt at exoneration: "Sam, I, all of us, want to help you feel better without taking that medicine. That's where Rose comes in. "

Sam screws up his eyes, says "Gotcha," and hunches over, elbows on knees, eyes on the floor.

I direct an upward nod to Rose to prompt her to get started with Sam but immediately feel like an exasperated detective passing the baton to my partner and decide to use my words, adding, "Rose, let's have you offer Sam your healing. But first, let's do some housekeeping." I get up and arrange Rose and Sam's chairs so they are facing each other straight on and move Londo's and mine back a couple of feet but leave them angled from their chairs. I definitely need to be here to observe the quality of Rose's psychotherapy (and not provide it myself) and am not sure how I feel about Londo's staying on but definitely want us to be as un-audience-like as possible.

Rose begins: "Sam, you got no energy, yeah?"

Sam: "Yes, mam. Dat de problem. Done gone."

Rose: "You know de doctor dinks you got depression, de sadness."

Sam: "Yes, mam, he done told me…. Dat's a good doctor coming all de way from America."

Rose: "Oh, yeah. Well, dem pills sometimes help de depression. But sometimes it take talking. I heal with de words. In Merica, dey call it derapy."

Sam: "What good talking do? Yeah, I sad. But I got sad dings. Sad life."

Here's where we need Sam to play the student and learn, making our schoolroom setting an apt touch for an orientation to CBT. I am just holding my breath to see how long Rose can hang in there as a teacher. Let's see it, Rose.

Rose: "Doctor told me you got sad dings—de war, your lady. I am sorry, so help me God. You do farm, yeah? Rice, yeah?"

Sam: "Yeah, dat don't make sad. So, what?"

Rose: "You got your own scythe?"

Sam, with impatience: "Yeah, you got rice needs harvesting? You need me scythe?"

Rose: "Is your scythe slicing de rice right now witout you?"

Sam, with even more impatience: "Dat's nonsense!"

Rose: "Sure is. It ain't no scythe witout you. It just wood and steel. It can't move, can't dink. Sadness de same."

Sam, waving a hand dismissively: "Can't farm rice wit sadness?!"

Rose: "No way you can. I sure do agree. But if a scythe ain't no scythe witout you, someting ain't sad witout you."

I am impressed, but is Sam?

Sam: "Yeah, dings don't cry, so? I'm not any fool."

Rose: "You sho not. But if something ain't sad witout you, it don't have to be so sad. Yeah, your lady up and leaves—everyone be sad if they have a heart. But not everyone who get sad have to lose energy. What dat go to do wit missing de lady?"

Sam sits back as much as his cramped seat allows and hanging his head back, slips his baseball cap over his face. But when he replaces his cap and sits back up, he does not bolt like Malike the wayward jackrabbit. This is going well.

Sam: "So, what does low energy have to do wit it?"

Rose: "It's what you dink dat matters. Sad ting and bad dinking and dere goes de energy."

Sam and Londo both seem to be lost in thought as Rose takes advantage of the silence to peel an orange. Docs shc know she's mixing metaphors? She passes around orange pieces to students and audience alike, and I am enjoying feeling like we are in nursery school. She just packaged the fundamental idea of CBT that how we think dictates our response to events around us in a metaphor befitting a someone who knew nothing of the psychotherapy and a lot about rice farming.

Londo looks like he thinks he's got it and decides to tag team the psychotherapy, asking Sam, "Hey, man, do you know what bad thinking you're doing?" Why did you have to jump in? Perfect question but I wish he hadn't asked it. First, people usually don't like being psychologically teamed up on; second, he may have just gotten farther ahead than Sam, who may still not have drunk the Kool Aid; and third, as impressed as I was with her so far, I want to see how Rose sees this through. I hope he just took the words right out of her mouth.

Sam says he does not know what bad thinking he's been doing and promises he goes to church. So, Rose astutely walks things back and asks, "Dis not about your faith…. Hey dere Sam, you get how bad dinking can make tings worse for you?"

Sam replies with a "I dink so" that is so unconvincing that Rose parries back with an equally unconvincing, "So, tell me what you dink about bad dinking?"

Sam gets the message and confesses confusion, earning a chalkboard lesson. Rose strides to the chalkboard and snatches up some chalk as though she had ordered these props in advance. She draws this picture on the board:

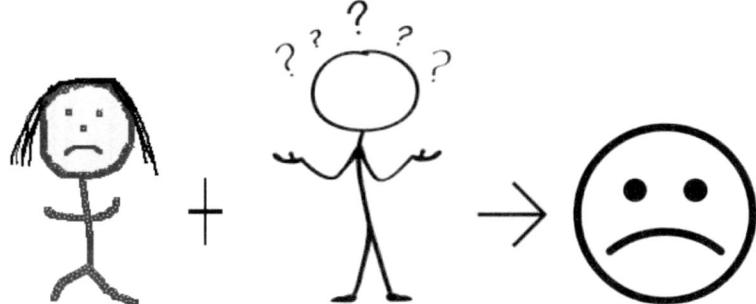

Rose: "Sam, over here, your lady, she unhappy and she does leave you. And way over here, you so sad. But right here in the middle, you see dose question marks? Yeah, you should be asking what you done did dat she do leave. No decent lady just leave. And any decent man, he be sad. But do see you all of dose question marks—you done gone ask too many questions. And den dey weigh you down. You question too much. And den you get tired... Dat's bad dinking."

Sam: "So, you done go and know my mind. Dat's what you do?"

Rose: "No, Sam. I can't tell you what you dink or what you feel. You do tell me."

Sam: "Well, if I already know my bad dinking, why do I need you?... Sorry, dat's rude."

Rose: "My friend, you ask good questions. Not rude... I give you de tools to help you figure out your dinking. So, how you done feel right now?

Sam: "I still tired, still sad. Dis talking not healing."

Rose: "We got to talk more. Not done. We just startin'. Today just a start."

Rose takes a paper out of a skirt pocket and places it in her lap, hunching over and mouthing to herself as she reads it. Then she looks up and asks Sam and asks, "When you look at your lady up here on the board, what you dink?"

"Ms. Rose, I don't even belong on de same board as Amara. Wipe me out. I ain't worth her," Sam laments. Then he dismisses the chalkboard with a wave and hunches back over his knees in retreat.

Rose pursues him, asking, "Well dere's your bad dinking—that you ain't worth your wife. Why you say dat?"

Sam stays hunched over but lifts his head to get another look at Rose before he sank further into the quicksand of his awfulness and pleaded, "You really wanna know?"

It's getting hotter in the classroom as the sun settles into its mid-afternoon power alley, preying on my historical penchant for drifting into sleep when watching someone else interview a patient. Londo has already succumbed, but I fight back. Sam talks with such earnest emotion , it is not hard to imagine the chalk and eraser coming to life and dancing Disney-like across the board, partnering to draw and erase scene after scene with the stick figures of Amara and Sam:

- Sam slouching in a chair in their tiny home, head in hand
- Sam staring out onto the street from the threshold of the home
- Amara touching Sam on his shoulder from behind
- Sam walking slump-shouldered down the street
- Sam at the bar, still slouching
- Four-year-old Mirlande crumpled over and crying next to her bicycle in the street
- Amara with Mirlande at Londo's practice
- Amara sitting on the edge of sleeping Mirlande's bed
- Sam sleeping outside with his back against the front of their home

"Dat's why I ain't worth it. If I listen to Amara and don't go... don't drink palm wine, dat never would happen. I no good husband no good daddy," Sam concludes. "Ain't no other way."

Sam's conviction snaps me out of my reverie like a judge's gavel. Rose lets it all hang in the air, lets Sam catch his breath, and lets the silence awaken Londo.

Rose: "Sam, what makes you dink you could do anyting 'bout Mirlande's tumble even if you were home?"

Sam: "Can't do noting from the bar...."

Rose: "True, true. But if you stay like Amara asks you, den what? Do you always watch Mirlande when she go on biking?"

Sam: "I should."

Rose: "Says who?"

Sam: "I dunno."

Rose: "I dunno, too. I done seen kids biking when we done arrived to town. No adults anywhere 'round."

Rose: "Has Mirlande ever fallen while you watched her?"

Sam: "Yes...."

Rose: "Well den I guess you being dere dat day and not out with the palm wine don't den promise her safety."

Sam: "I guess you make de point."

Rose: "See dat? Dat's your bad dinking."

Rose stops for a moment, and I am guessing she's deciding where to go next while letting the jury of one consider the evidence. Now she asks Sam how Mirlande got her bike.

Sam: "I bought it for her."

Rose: "Musta cost you. How you do dat?"

Sam: "I just did. Daddies do dat."

Rose: "Sure, but how you do dat?"

And with that prodding the chalkboard comes alive again:

- Mirlande sitting in the street watching kids bicycling
- Amara and Sam talking
- Sam unloading cargo from a ship under the moonlight
- Sam milking cows in the sunlight
- Sam and Mirlande sitting together on a bus
- Sam and Mirlande talking to a clerk at a store
- Sam and Mirlande smiling on another bus with a bicycle in the aisle
- Mirlande bicycling with her friends

Sam comes to no conclusion of his own this time, but Rose does: "You done mean you work two extra jobs for months, take a bus to the big city, buy your girl a beautiful bicycle, put a smile on your precious girl's face, and you not wort someting as a daddy? Not wort a lot as a daddy?"

Sam admits she's right, to which she declares, "Now we got some good dinking."

Rose is done. If this were baseball, now she would flip her bat and circle the bases with face down, not even needing to watch her homerun sail out of the park or Sam run home ahead of her. At the least, it feels like she and Sam should join hands and take a bow. Rather than clapping for either scenario, I ask Sam, "So, Sam how do you feel?"

"Well, doctor I do feel good. I do feel like I done went to de hospital," Sam offers.

"Sam, you see that's how healing happens with words. Who needs medicine that stuffs you up?" I declare.

Chapter 16

Harold P. Doll

Before Berko get up, I untie his wrist from de arm of de bench. Then I done try to wake him up, but he no budge. Do I have to do everyting for you, even do de waking for you?

"Berko, Berko, wake up, you!" I shout when tapping de shoulder don't do.

You dink sleeping in de church pews would make you want to leap up de moment you could, but dat only happens in de middle of de night, when we get into a row over his wanderin'. But never, ever in de morning wit de rest of us, when we get into anoter row. And dis mornin', we need to go see the doctor from Merica.

Dat boy done spend tree weeks, I dink, in dat hospital. I wish he don't need to see doctor never again, but Doctor Mary done say he can't stop de medicine. And no doctor, no medicine 'cause we got no money to just walk to de pharmacy and say "Give me dat. Here de money for it." Dat's for de rich folks, dose Buzzards who can swoop in and buy what dey need. Be deir own doctor and bank. But I bet dey don't need no government psychitrist, don't even need any psychitrist. Dey got it all.

Berko yell back, "Ife, me wife, I so tired. Let me be. We got nuttin to do."

Unseen: Field Notes of a Global Psychiatrist
Craig L. Katz
Copyright © 2025 Jenny Stanford Publishing Pte. Ltd.
ISBN 978-981-5129-42-7 (Hardcover), 978-1-003-56767-7 (eBook)
www.jennystanford.com

"Berko, we sure 'nough do got somethin' to do—you go to see de doctor, an American doctor. Dey check de medicine you on," I remind him.

I met de doctor last night when Londo's wife and I made him and his team dinner. I can't believe he come all de way from America, and he has to eat de dinner at a school desk and den sleep in a classroom. At least Londo had de ingredients to make my special porridge. And at least dey had cots at de school from de war when teachers gotta stay a lot because of fightin' on de road.

Mention of de doctor is as good as a rooster, and Berko get up and rubs de wrist. But tank de Lord, leaves it at dat. We go to de river to freshen up and brush de teeth and then come back to say our mornin' prayers, but dat just upset him. We be kneeling at de altar, but he cry like a baby and falls face down when we get to de part about peace. When get past dat, we den eat some bread and leftover porridge. It not hot but it still be good, dat's how good it is. His porridge is de extra special kind—I done grind up his medicine from Doc Mary and put it in, but not every day dat easy with just bread or fruit. You can't make a medicine sandwich or pretend dat a pit for eatin'.

I don't remember if we wait for de doctor or go to de doctor but don't want to make him wait. So, I smooth over Berko's hair, and we go.

"Ife, I don't want to take dat medicine today. What if de doctor find out?" Berko, my innocent man, asks.

"It OK sweetie, it OK," I assure him wit my fingers crossed.

A dog go runnin' by, and Berko starts to run wit him. De dog go faster, with dat tongue hanging out so far and flapping around so much I done dink he looks like one of tose airplanes 'bout to take off. Don't know where Berko find tat energy when he spends de days nodding off. Now, I got to remind him we on our way to de doctor— "Hey, there's only doctor but lots a dogs where dat came from!"

We go to de school, and Londo's wife, she dere already, settin' up coffee and some breakfast bread and jam and boiled eggs on de teacher's desk in one classroom. There's an empty cot with de mosquito net hangin' from a single hook on de ceiling, and it's wide open. She says de doctor done gone for a walk around de town. Maybe I need to take Berko's medicine, because I see dat and I dink that look like a cocoon done give birth to de doctor. De others, de healer lady, Rose, and Johnny de driver are in other classrooms, and I hear dem stirrin' like dey gettin' up to de smell of de coffee.

I chitchat with Londo's wife and den with de others when dey come in to eat while Berko draws pictures on de chalkboard. Den de doctor comes back and says he sorry we been waitin'. He had not met Berko yet and introduces himself proper like a good doctor.

Doctor eats real fast and asks us to sit down into de student chairs to talk. De healer comes, too, but Johnny goes out. We in a circle.

"So, Berko, tell me how you are?" de doctor asks.

"I'm ok, danks, sir," he responds.

"I'm a psychiatrist, and I heard you were just at the psychiatric hospital. Why did you need to go to the hospital?" de doctor asks.

"I dunno, doc. Ife, she say I need to go, and I done listen to my wife. Doc Mary, she agree, says I need to get better sleep," Berko says.

"Did she tell you what your condition is?" the doctor asks.

"Yes, sir. She done say my mind goes too much. Dat's why I can't sleep," Berko offered.

"So, how are you now?" de doctor asks.

"Ahh… I don't like Harold P. Doll. It no good," Berko explained, but doctor looks very confused.

"Doctor, he done mean de medicine Doc Mary prescribe," I jump in. "Dat's what he calls it, but I dink it's not right. Here de bottle."

"Ah, you are taking what we call in America, haloperidol. I hope it's helping you sleep?" doctor says wit hope.

"I can't sleep. Sometin' keeps comin' in de night and tie me up. Some demon. Harold P. Doll can't help wit dat. But Ife, she protect me," Berko explains and reaches for my hand.

"I am really sorry to hear that. It must be very frightening, but you have a good lady looking after you. Do you take your medicine every day?" doctor asks.

"I sure do, 'cause Doc Mary she done say so," Berko lies.

I ask de doctor to step outside so I can explain de facts. We go to de porch of de school.

"We left de hospital last week, and he be better. Still talkin' nonsense but not acting it so much. Dey give us de pills and say never to stop 'em. But not sure how we can get 'em or pay for 'em since we don't live near de hospital. I dink we have enough for one month. And it not true dat he take it every day. He don't like it. Says it makes him tired, gives him headache, makes him feel not right. He say, 'Dat Harold, he ain't no doll.' So, sometimes I get him to take it and sometimes I mix it into de food," I say so quick it's like I am tellin' on him to daddy. Deep breath.

"And please dear Lord forgive me. Dat demon he talk about dat tie him up? Dat me. Maybe he tired but not at de right time. He keep getting' up and moseying away. So, when he done get up, I act de hero and untie him. If it's de middle of de night, I watch until he fall back and den I tie him again," I say just as quick 'cause now I am tellin' on me.

The doctor forgives me. He says, "Ife, you're no demon. You are a loving wife doing all you can for Berko. Who knows what would happen to him without you trying to get him to take the medicine or stopping him from wandering in the night? I have seen people back home do less with more, but you do more with less. "

Now Berko comes on out and say, "Doctor, are you done wit me? I gotta go."

I tell Berko, "Berko, the good doctor, he not done. Where you gotta go!?" Berko goes right back in.

"Ife, I had a chance to speak to Doc Mary about Berko, and you are right he needs to be on medicine all the time. Do you know what his diagnosis is?" he asks me.

I say back, "I guess I don't know de fancy name, but I do know de game. He scared when nothing is dere; he talk nonsense; he cry over little dings. He done see what he dinks but needs to dink what he sees."

"I could not describe it any better. But just so you know, the name doctors give for all of that is schizophrenia," the doctor explains.

"Well, that good to know because my family don't want us back. Dat's why we are back here, sleepin' in de church. We went home after de hospital, but dey turn us away just like before de hospital. So, we come back here to Londo de healer hopin' he can help. He find a way for us to stay at de church and help wit food. But I don't know how long dis can keep goin'. Maybe dey be okay if dey knew about dis fancy name," I wonder aloud.

De doctor tell me dat he has some medicine on him better than Harold P. Doll. He brought it from de States but did not know if he could use it because it's only enough for one person. But now he done find dat person, and we go back in.

De doctor tells Berko, "Sorry to make you wait, Berko. So, I know Harold P. Doll has been bothering you. I have a medicine I brought from America that I think should be better. It's called Leridone."

Berko, he say nothin' and stands up. He stretches his arms up high and look up to de ceiling. We all wait while he does dis. De healer looks confused, and de doctor just looks. I see him do tings like this before and just wait. When Berko sit down he announces dat he will take the medicine.

De doctor gives me de bottle and tells Berko he can start with one-half pill every day and can go up to a whole one if it don't bother him. He has to take it every day, and doctor will try to get us more from de States before it runs out.

Den De doctor steps to de door and calls for Johnny. Dey whisper to one another, and I wonder what's happenin' until the doctor comes back and says he wants to go meet my family and explain Berko's problem. I dank him so much for dis idea from God and ask Johnny if he knows how to get there.

Den Johnny says to de doctor, "What about de healer, Londo. He coming?"

De doctor says dat not needed—he can talk to de family like a doctor. But den Johnny, he say, "Remember Malike?" and dis mean something to de doctor 'cause he said, "Ah, yes. I better not do this alone." But when nobody can find Londo, I say, "What about Rose? She a healer," and de doctor again says, "Ah, yes."

I got hope and before we all go in de big van, I go get our tings from de church. Soon as Johnny turns de key, de van roars and Berko snores. He sleeps sideways-like against de window, but my window ain't no pillow. I can't recollect de last time I been in an auto, and I feel like a princess bein' driven and watchin' de world from up high. I wave as we go, and I'm likin' de view from de other side of dings for once.

We get to my parents' farm and everyone stand around wonderin' what next while I go find daddy in de fields. He greet me wit a hug and a "you finally made de right decision." But when I break de news dat Berko is waiting back at de house, he just go walking off into de rice field searchin' for answers. But I yell dat a doctor from America came wit us and wants to speak to him, and we go walkin' back real quiet.

It's big news in de village when a shiny government van show up, and it's de newest of news when it brings along a white doctor. So, after introductions, our team gotta make its way through de neighbors gatherin' round and follows my father into de house. Mommy hugs me and den rushes to get de guests tea. Daddy, doctor, Berko, and me done sit in de living room while Johnny and Rose stand around.

Daddy plays like de judge while doctor talks:

Doctor: "Sir, please excuse our barging into your home like this, but I felt it was important."

Daddy: "Please, doctor, do go on."

Doctor: "Your son-in-law has a serious medical condition that requires medication. He's gotten a lot better since being in the hospital, but if he stops taking it, then he will get sick again. He respects you, and I am hoping you can help."

Berko: "Hey, I do take de medicine!"

Daddy: "Doctor, I know Berko, he not right. And I betcha he done got a medical problem you know mo' about dan me. But dese people, dey done dink he possessed...."

In America, you got privacy, but here we got neighbors. They be standin' around de livin' room, standin' in de doorway, and hangin' through de windows like dey been invited. Dey de jury, and when daddy say dis, they start their murmuring until Rose, she says, "Hush, de doctor talkin'!"

Daddy: "...And if they dink he possessed, dey won't work my farm or buy my rice. I got a business to run and a family dat done need it to eat."

Doctor now looks around the room as he speaks, saying, "Berko has a problem of the mind. We don't know what causes it, but we do know medicine helps it. I have brought a new medicine from America that should be even better than the medicine from the hospital."

And someone wit no manners challenges de doctor, "You got enough of dat medicine for de whole town 'cause we'll all need it real soon!?"

Doctor says it don't work dat way, but dere's just more murmuring as daddy sits there wishing he weren't sitting there. Suddenly Johnny pipes up: "Hey, it's not like dat. I been workin' at the psychitry hospital for fifteen years, and I never get mind problems!" Dat quiets dings for a tic of de clock until someone shouts, "Don't be so sure!" and there's laughter dat makes me wanna cry.

Doctor raises his voice and asks, "Does anyone here have arthritis?" And when a few people raise de hand, he goes on, "Well that's a problem of the bones and the joints. This is no different except it is in the mind, a different part of the body. For both problems, you see a healer or a doctor and get help."

People seem to be dinking dis over when Rose steps forward and rings out, "Is anyone among you sick?" and den pauses and looks around before going on: "Let dem call the elders of de church to pray over dem and anoint dem with oil in de name of God. Dat's from de good Lord's Bible, Book of James... Chapter 5, Verse 14."

It gets real silent, and den Rose asks, "Doctor, what is de name of de medicine for Berko?"

He says, "It's called Leridone."

Rose asks doctor to hold up the bottle of Leridone for all to see and den concludes, "Dat dere Leridone, you all done see it? That Leridone is de oil for anointin' Berko in de name of God."

Well, Rose, she done settle dat, and de people start pulling away like de flood waters. But daddy, he sit dere and still trying to settle it for himself. He asks de doctor, "So, what we do now?"

De doctor answers, "Well, we see how this new medicine goes for Berko, and we help make sure he takes it. And if you can give him work and keep him productive, that sure will help, too."

Daddy still lookin' real serious and asks, "But what if Berko does not take your medicine? And what if it don't work so well?"

De doctor says it straight: "Then he goes back to the hospital."

And Berko says, "I do take de medicine!"

Chapter 17

Story Lines

Dr. Juma resigned as director of the psychiatric hospital just weeks after I left. When I rang her on WhatsApp to discuss how to get more Leridone to Berko, she announced that she finally agreed to join the faculty of a new medical school just over the border in their wealthier neighbor. "I'm going to be just like you, professor!"

Mental Mary will mostly be teaching primary care medicine but was also asked to help with psychiatric education, undoubtedly a cost-effective bundle of expertise for the fledgling school. When she vented to me about Dr. Toussaint's over-reliance on her, that was clearly the tip of a tropical iceberg. I think the calvary in the form of me and my ideas had just come too late to rescue Mary from burnout, while my inadvertent role modeling as a medical educator did. Good for her, not for her country. As I sit here on my professorial throne at the medical student clinic, who am I to judge?

Without Dr. Juma, there was no obvious replacement for my in-country liaison, but "this" does not work without one. Remember that Wheel of Global Mental Health I mentioned earlier? It's mostly made up of elements that consider "their" needs, resources, and aspirations and "our" resources and aspirations. But the in-country liaison completes the circle. The Wheel stops revolving without them, which is precisely why I had stopped off and had some PBJ with Dr. Toussaint while in-country. Ideally, Mary's replacement

Unseen: Field Notes of a Global Psychiatrist
Craig L. Katz
Copyright © 2025 Jenny Stanford Publishing Pte. Ltd.
ISBN 978-981-5129-42-7 (Hardcover), 978-1-003-56767-7 (eBook)
www.jennystanford.com

would be Dr. Toussaint, as the senior physician in their public health system and Mary's boss, but if not, he would assume responsibility for designating her successor.

I had written to Dr. Toussaint immediately about the situation, and he emailed back within minutes. "Maybe you would like to replace her?" It was impossible to gather his tone, but his speedy response conveyed gravity. It was not the first time I had received such a simultaneously tantalizing and fantastical proposition.

I wrote back ("If only I could!") and asked if I could rely on him as my point person to follow up on my long-term ideas for plugging their mental health gap that I had discussed with Mary before I left. Dr. Toussaint replied with a nearly immediate "Of course, let's be in touch." But when he did not even ask what those ideas were, I had a sense this was an empty promise, and I was right: I have now been waiting three weeks for his reply about getting Berko his medication.

As I now think about it, I realize we have never told our liaisons they are our liaisons—never offered them a title, even an adjunct faculty appointment at our medical school, let alone some extra pay. We may operate on a shoestring budget wherein most of our doctors donate their time, but that budget surely looks like Cinderella's slipper to our partners. I know people like Mary are in it for the good of their patients and communities, but formalizing or incentivizing their relationship with us can only help. Right now, Mental Mary could have been both an assistant professor (at an American medical school!) and director of the psychiatric hospital all at once.

Well, Mary may be gone and Dr. Toussaint MIA, but Londo remains on the case, and I have never thought in all my teaching or planning that a healer could be our liaison and still do not. Someone like Londo lacks the country-wide influence and connections that are important, not even to other healers, as I only know of one country where traditional healers are organized into a national organization. Someone like him also lacks the resources. And so it was that it took Molly and Power Up to come to the rescue once more and get Londo a smartphone and a wireless hotspot so he could video chat with Mary about Berko. But I think I need to add Deputy Liaison to the Wheel and offer Londo the inaugural position.

Since Mary left, I have been filling in for her on the other end of the video chat with Londo. Berko and Ife have been making the full-day trek on foot to see Londo every two weeks since I left. Her father excuses him from work for the two days it takes to go, stay over in the church, and walk back the next day. Berko's been taking the Leridone. He calls it "Londone" and says it doesn't bother him. When I ask if it helps him, he says he's been sleeping well. He also mentions he's not been getting tied up anymore and when I attempt to peer deeper into his mind and ask him to explain what he thinks that has to do with the medication, he simply says, "Londone, it just done help." When I ask him if his mind still goes too fast, he usually says something like, "Don't dink so, but you gotta ask Ife."

Ife's reports have generally been positive, too. It's been less of a struggle to get Berko to take his medication. And with him in earshot, she has generally reported that the nights have been "free of de issues" and needs to say no more. She also has been reporting that he's been making much more sense, so much so that her father has allowed him to resume driving the truck, although he can't spare it for their trips to Londo. How did she put it one time…. "Less dinkin', more truckin'." At one point, an unfamiliar healer came and performed a fire ritual in front of their house at the apparent behest of some of their neighbors. But that seemed to put an end to any obvious community dissension about Berko living there, as I am sure his improvement has, too.

When I see Ife, it looks like a weight has been lifted off of her shoulders. But in that vein, it looks like Berko has gotten a lot heavier. They say cameras put on weight, but I wish it were just that. I fear he's developing some of the metabolic problems characteristic of Leridone. I know there were some real problems with how I have gone about this. "Londone" can definitely cause significant weight gain and at least temporary bumps in cholesterol readings or blood sugar, this is at a time when problems like heart disease, high blood pressure, and diabetes are already becoming rampant in the developing world as historic gains are made against the more traditional specter of infectious diseases. But unlike how I would proceed with most patients here in America, I gave Berko the medication without discussing the risks. In fact, I told him it would not bother him as much, when in fact it could well have over-sedated him, even if this were less likely than the haloperidol.

Maybe I am turning this over in my mind more than I need to, but it was not like there was an alternative medication with a better side-effect profile I could offer. I did not know if he would understand. I was also desperate to help and did not want anything to get in the way, even if I am sure Ife would have understood and probably still have blessed it given how desperate she was. I have no doubt Berko was better off trying than not trying the Leridone, but I wonder if wanting to play hero too much affected how I presented it to him. Did I wind up playing at God instead of returning home with a knapsack full of Leridone and empty hand sanitizer bottles?

And of course, the other real problem is that I had no clear path for assuring Berko's supply going forward and still don't. Leridone, as a new brand-new-to-market medication, costs over $1,500 per month, which may make my dropping it into Berko's life an ultimately outlandish move; pharmaceutical representatives will not be able to "sample" me indefinitely on his behalf. But many of our psychiatric medications are available as very affordable generic versions, an increasing number of which have been incorporated into the World Health Organization's model formulary for countries, known as the Essential Medication List. Figuring out what it would take for a low-income country to reliably stock the eighteen or so psychiatric medications on the EML is a quixotic puzzle. Ever idealistic if not masochistic, we're actually trying to solve it as I write in another country. But that foretells a future for dreamers. For now, Berko, Sam, and their countrymen are left with just two or three of those medications as options.

Risk-benefit inheres in every medical decision, and I have come to think that even if the Leridone runs out, at least I gave Berko and Ife three months of relative peace they otherwise would have lacked and hopefully shown her father and especially their town Berko's problem can be seen as a medical problem, not necessarily one of spiritual possession. Of course, whatever befalls Berko or Sam, theirs remains a country without a functioning mental health system for all. Funders for our trips inevitably want to hear what our "outcomes" are and ask an understandable if somewhat infuriating question—"How many people did you serve?" Two will not cut it, but having only started the job, I cannot yet lay claim to the millions who populate the country or the likely tens to hundreds of thousands who need psychiatric care of some sort.

As anyone who's undergone mental health treatment knows, psychiatric recovery usually takes weeks to months or even longer and often entails years of ongoing care rather than an outright cure. Global mental health is even more so a long-term project. Maybe I left my diplomatic tact back at the Ministry of Health, but it seems to me that many people with the money that could easily help us bridge the global mental health gap (one estimate says that it would take around $USD 1 billion per year to hire enough mental health professionals) think that because their contribution can be quantified so must mine.

I cannot wait until what we achieve is so big it should be counted, but it seems neither can a lot of funders. They repeatedly steer away from mental health, even in the United States. Do they not see the need or, for reasons best left to Freud, not want to see it? I admit I am wary when "we need more money!" is the proposed solution to a problem, but the idealism and all too frequent voluntarism of global mental health professionals cannot alone close the mental health gap.

My attention to Berko also meant operating, unsustainably, at the individual level when my patient was supposed to be in his country. But I just cannot stop being a doctor when I am being a public health professional. On the other hand, new treatments and new approaches always start with observations in individual cases, and here I have helped craft a miniature system for Berko and Ife that incorporates Molly and Power Up as funders, Londo as a partner in healing, initially Mary and for now myself as a supervisor, and the manufacturer of Leridone. If it works, maybe it can be replicated on a not-so-miniature level for the other Berko's out there, maybe starting with some or all of the patients at the psychiatric hospital. Maybe this is the start of a system of utilizing traditional healers as what you might call mental health ambassadors to shift needlessly long hospital care into the community.

Rose may make the point of starting every journey with a footstep even better. I was very impressed by Rose. She seemed like a natural at CBT and a person for whom healing of any stripe came naturally. And Sam really took well to his session with her. I went back to the bank that is Molly and was able to secure payment for Rose at the same rate she was paid in the research study to meet with Sam weekly for ten more sessions, a pretty typical number for CBT for depression.

I was also able to connect Rose with one of our CBT mavens, Dr. Arhoski, to provide her with some long-distance supervision. That's been happening by videoconferencing about weekly at the Power Up office where they have a computer and internet for Rose to use. She also uses the office to conduct remote CBT with Sam—on his end, he goes to Londo and uses his smartphone. Here the mini mental health system of Rose, Molly and Power Up, and Dr. Arhoski operate on behalf of Sam.

Now, from the research publication on the CBT study in which Rose participated, we know 14 other CBT therapists were trained. I wanted to find them and pilot a CBT for depression program at Dr. Ali's hospital, probably starting with a few of them in Dr. Robinson's clinic. Since the in-country coordinator was sadly no longer alive, I emailed the head of the Global CBT Project to find out their plans and try to get the CBT therapists' names and any viable contact information they might have so many years later.

We spoke on the phone, and the project director told me that their private grant funding for following up the study began to dry up while the Ministry of Health showed zero interest in picking it up on their tab, even before the outbreak of the virus in the country. I proposed to do what I could to revive things and asked if they could give me the information about the CBT trainees. They told me they would need to check with their research oversight board because the trainees were considered subjects in the study just like their clients and therefore their identities may need to remain confidential for ethical reasons. I am hoping that is the issue and that it's a surmountable one and that they are not just being territorial. I am still waiting to hear back from them. If that does not pan out, we can always train people in CBT ourselves, even if it means slowing things down. We've done it. In the meanwhile, I emailed a copy of their publication to Molly so she can download and print it for Rose. I opted not to chide the project director for not doing this themselves.

I have to admit that my drive-by at Father Reginald's compound yielded nothing comparable to Berko or Sam for helping Amadu and his peers. As most of them are still kids, if not in body then in minds stunted from too much violence and too little love, we need child and adolescent mental health expertise and trauma expertise, while either alone is a highly specialized and scarce resource unto itself. And this is all the more so the case since we have our own shortage of child mental health professionals here in America. I have such a hard time recruiting them to work with our global mental health program because they're flooded with their own work. Amadu and the orphanage are a tall order, and I have for now opted to pluck the lower-hanging fruit of the CBT program, but they're on my list. My wife's a child psychiatrist who worked overseas even before I did, and I may even just have to start there in literal mom-and-pop fashion.

Training CBT, child/adolescent, trauma, or other types of lay psychotherapists (there are by some counts over 400 types of psychotherapy, but few so universal as CBT and many that seem like variations on a theme) is not just about addressing mental health. It can have an economic benefit. Poverty contributes to mental health problems, but mental health problems can drag people down into poverty. If you make a community mentally healthier, you make it more productive, an important observation for those for whom numbers count.

Productivity also matters for much of the world, even in places where you will find people who cannot count, as most cultures tends to consider mental health (if it considers mental health) to be about how well someone contributes to their family and community and shun the West's emphasis on the individual and their experience. If you are interested here's how the World Health Organization defines mental health, one that conspicuously leaves out something all of my patients, and I think, all Americans hold dearly, happiness: "Mental health can be conceptualized as a state of well-being in which the individual realizes his or her own abilities, can cope with the normal stresses of life, can work productively and fruitfully, and is able to make a contribution to his or her community."

And if nothing else, if you train people like Rose to be psychotherapists, even if they need supervision and experience to really become adept at it, they now have a skill and potential new job likely far more remunerative than selling fruit so long as someone will pay. Right now, of course, people in most of the world do not even give a second thought to the value of fruit, whereas they do not even know enough to give an initial thought to mental health, let alone attribute value to and pay for it. We have a lot of awareness-building to do, something psychiatrists and other mental health professionals tend to be awful at, instead preferring that people who are not "psychologically minded" not waste their time. They want good patients, but the world needs good healers. Calling all mental health professionals ready to cultivate, not demand, psychological mindedness!

They should also be ready to work atop a quivering house of cards. Molly had to resign from her overseas posting to return home to be with her mother, Sylvia, as her manic-depression continued to wreak havoc in her life. She got arrested for punching out a cashier who asked her to bag her own groceries, and now she has legal problems on top of everything else. Molly was kind enough to text me about her decision, if you can call it that when you have no real choice, and then emailed to introduce me to her successor at Power Up's in-country office. I never actually met Molly in person, but we had developed a nice working relationship. And Power Up's funds have repeatedly been an essential ingredient in arranging things on behalf of Berko and Sam. It's worrisome—but I have always told myself and the occasional patient that I am paid to worry so they don't have to.

Mary's gone, Molly's gone, Leridone's nearly gone. One of my students, after completing a course I teach on global mental health in which I spell out all the challenges that seem to define it, crowned me the most determined person in the world to be trying to make it a mentally healthier place. But I am not the most determined person in the world. People like Mary, Ife, Nurse Providence, Johnny, Father Reginald, Virginia here in the U.S.—they have to live all of this and need every bit of determination. I walk alongside of the most determined people in the world, the top award for which should go to Sam.

Chapter 18

Sam III

"I can help," I do say wit hand raised high. De Power Up people done hold anotha meetin' and dis time I make it.

"Thanks. Please sign the volunteer list when it comes to you and be sure to include your cell phone. Anyone else? Just to recap, we want to hold groups for former Bustards to meet with widows of former Buzzards and heal the wounds from the war. We call these healing circles. They will be really powerful."

I don't know how to write my name, but I do go up to de lady after and give my name. She's not Miss Molly, who done gone back to de States, and I don't know her name. But she seem nice. I am glad I finally go to one of their meet-ups, but I do wish Miss Molly could see I finally gone and came.

It's a nice cool night, and I decide to stop by de food shack to see my friends and have dinner, somethin' I also not done in a long time. Dis time, I eat good but no more palm wine, even when my friends gotta always say somethin' about somethin'. Dey been drinkin' so much I don't even tink dey missed me. Why should dey care if I don't join de party and drink?

I been getting' my energy back, danks to Rose. After dat first meetin' the good doctor and Miss Molly done set it up so Rose meet with me for more healin' sessions every week. Dey also call dem 'pointments in America and said one healin' 'pointment of dat CBT is

Unseen: Field Notes of a Global Psychiatrist
Craig L. Katz
Copyright © 2025 Jenny Stanford Publishing Pte. Ltd.
ISBN 978-981-5129-42-7 (Hardcover), 978-1-003-56767-7 (eBook)
www.jennystanford.com

good but not lastin' and dey were right. I felt real good after dat first time but it didn't last more than a day. Not sure why dat is, but dey de healin' people, not me.

It felt like a long time until de next meetin' wit Rose, and it was not de same. They had me do it from de phone at Londo's by video. Rose was in de capital. It was okay, but de video kept stoppin', and I felt real rude havin' to keep ask her to repeat herself 'cause de sound not much better. De phone done need more energy dan me! Plus, how does healin' work over de phone anyways?

We done got smart and figured out a way for me to go visit Rose. Londo, he gave me some plantain from de farm, and I went and sold it wit' Rose. She don't mind a little less business 'cause she got a blessed soul, she does. De money I make, I give half to Londo and keep de other half for myself for de bus rides to get dere and home. If you're countin, you might wonder how I paid for dat first bus ride in before I even sell de plantain?

Well, I been workin' extra in de rice fields. My energy get better just in time for harvestin' time, and I done promise my boss to work hard. He knew I was not de same last harvest, but he done just let it go. When I am in de fields now, my scythe got de power back again, more dan any of dose torches from Ms. Molly will ever have.

Well, I'm lost in my head dinkin' about all dis, and dat my friends notice. De say, "Hey Sam, you don't drink but are you drunk? Where are you, man? De good Lord's earth to Sam: Come in Sam?!" Well, dat's enough for me , and I just wave them off and leave and go sit in a chair outside my home and dink a much as I like.

It's much better to spend time dinkin' when you not dinkin' bad. And oh, Lord, Rose she been workin' wit me on those thoughts over and over. God done bless her. After we sell all of our fruit, we go to de Power Up office and get into de CBT. Each time she starts by checkin' on my mood by showin' me pictures of faces that go from cryin' sad to smilin' real bright. Den we plan de session—can't say I ever really plan anytin' in my life like dat before. You can't just take tings as dey come if you want to get somethin' out of it. Den we do it and den she give me homework to do, 'cause dat's what you do in CBT.

But dat was a problem. I can't read, can't write, and so how could I do homework? We get smart again. Instead of writin' it, I would call Rose's cell phone and leave a message, and we would review my messages at each 'pointment. The two homeworks I remember are 'bout activities and automatic thoughts. I say dose words real clear because Rose done say it real important to get it straight.

Wit activities, you keep track of everyting you do 'cause what you do can make you feel tings. I dink de real way to do dat is to track everyting every day all de time. But poor Rose's phone can't handle so many calls from me. So we do it for a day here and a day here, 'about every week. De activity log done show I don't do 'nough—it be either farmin' or nothin'. And when you do nothin', your mind don't do nothin'—it get busy, and den you start dinkin' dings too much. So, going to dat Power Up meetin' or eatin' dinner at de dinner shack (witout palm wine) wit de friends are de product of lookin' at what I do and figurin' out what I don't do.

When Rose first told me 'bout automatic thoughts, I done tink she mean car thoughts, because I done tink she meant "automobile," which make no sense because what dat mean? But when I got it dat we be monitorin' the thoughts I have, I remembered back to de first session we had—we be watchin' me for bad dinkin'. Now, dat's how been spendin' most of our time. My homework usually go like dis: When I get sad or worried, I am supposed to say to myself, "What's de situation and what am I dinkin' about it"? Then, I decide on some action—what am I goin' to do to feel better? So, each time I get sad, I done go and leave Rose a message, sayin' what bad feelin' I had, what de situation is, what my thought was, and what I done do about it. I guess she write dese dings down the proper way, and we go over dem next time. Dey are a lot and so, Rose asks me if I remember one dat I want to start wit. Den we keep making bad dinkin' into good dinkin'.

I learned 'nough from Rose that I dink I even helped Miss Molly wit it. I was leavin' de Power Up office after a 'pointment when Miss Molly came to me and done tell me she was leavin' de country 'cause of family problems. I danked her so much and while I did dat, she just start cryin' and cryin' like de typhoon floods gone and come again. I went runnin' back to Rose in de office we use, but she was talkin' on her phone and I was 'fraid to interrupt her. So, dinkin' I just can't leave dat poor girl cryin' out there by herself for so long, I go running back out and say she should try sittin'. Den I go to dat fancy upside-down water bottle they have and push de button for some water and give it to her, like I am fillin' her backup from all de lost tears like my ma always done said.

She 'pologizes to me, saying she should not be cryin' in front of me, it's not proper wit a client. I am 'bout to speak to dat when she done say, "It's just that everything's ruined now. Everything I worked for."

Now, I saw her bad dinkin as clear as dat water and said to her, "Miss Molly, you go ahead and be sad about leavin'. I do understand. But don't you go on dinkin everyting is ruined. Dat not true, just not true. I dink Rose would call dat 'black and white' dinkin'."

She gave me a look dat I thought meant I had gone too far, but den she said, "But how do you know? How do you know it's not all ruined?" And she wasn't insultin' me—she really wanted to know what I saw.

So, I said, "Miss Molly, just look at me, look at me here wit Rose. We're goin' keep doin' this after you leave, and I am goin' keep getting better 'cause of you."

Well, den de typhoon of tears done stop and Miss Molly danked me. She was still sad, but in de right way when you have to say goodbye.

Now, here's a story of how Rose de CBT healer helped me. Amara, she just don't answer my calls. I call and call and no answer. So, den I stopped leavin' messages and den I stopped callin'. First problem was an activity problem—whenever I felt like callin' and was missin' her so much, I would look at her picture up on de wall and just sit there like dat, dinkin' I miss her and feelin' bad. Dat means I am sittin' alone and dat just make de problem worse. So, when I feel like dat, if I don't call, den I need go out—go to de fields and work or go play cards wit friends. Do somethin'.

Now, second problem was my bad dinkin'. When she don't call me, my automatic thought was, "She ain't love me no more." Dat's all I could dink. And oh, how it hurt de soul. In a 'pointment, Rose done ask me to dink about dis and to dink if there could be any otha reasons why Amara don't call me. We done sit there dinkin' of what else. Maybe her parents are tellin' her not to call me, and she wants to be a good daughter. Maybe what I said in my messages was de problem, 'cause I was actin' real angry and shoutin' into de phone. So, maybe she was 'fraid to call me.

And now, here de one that really helped me dink a lot different—if she really didn't love me, she wouldn't care. She'd talk to me to just tell me to leave her alone and stop callin'. Maybe, then, she was hurtin' too much to call me, AND she was hurtin' too much 'cause she done still loved me. Rose, she made no promises dat any of dis were true, but de point was dat dinkin' Amara don't love me no more is just one way it could be. That's real smart, and it was a relief to see dings don't have to be what you been dinkin'.

Rose said dat it was possible my not callin' and not tryin' no more could have hurt Amara even more. So, first I done go and started callin' Amara again. Second, I don't just hang up when she don't pick up de phone. Tird, I leave sweet messages, not angry ones. It was like, "Amara, I miss you so much. I wish I could talk to you and to de girls." And you know what, one day she done pick up de phone!

After she put de girls on, I made my case to my lady, saying, "Amara, I don't drink de palm wine no more. I done stop."

"Dat's good, Sam, dat's good," she said, but dat's all.

"Amara, I miss you and de girls. I try real hard to be a good husband and good fatha," I keep goin' and hopin'. But when dat gets de silent treatment, I done tell her 'bout my derapy.

Bu, dis is what she say back: "Sammy, yo' wife and girls done leave you and you learnin' yo ABCs and doin' yo homework. What's dat?? Are you a schoolboy or a husband and father?!"

I said, first no it's "CBT," not "ABC," although I done forget what C, B, and T done mean. And second, if it's like de school, it's school about de self, to be a better self. Not just some book learnin'. And it's de healing sessions with Rose de healer that made de difference, I done tell her, not de homework, which ain't like doin' your times tables anyway.

Then she said, "Now you tellin' me you try to win back yo wife by seein' anotha woman?" And dat ended de call I been waitin' forever to have.

After dat, I got real bad again, real weak and like I never saw Rose. My bad dinkin' for dat next 'pointment was like dis: "I can't do anythin' right." Rose, she done make me dink about de dings I do right in my family, like even de sweet messages I left Amara dat made her call me back. Or like dat bike I bought for Mirlande. Den we talk about how I act after dis. I done decide not to call Amara again 'cause what's de point? Rose, she tell me that my choice is both good and bad. Good 'cause it sounds like tellin' Amara dis stuff on de phone don't work, she not listen' right. Some dings best done said in person. But not callin' no more means not communicatin' and dat's bad. Nothin' get better like dat. We decide I need to go visit Amara so she can see me and hear me. I feel ready.

Amara's parents done live 'bout a four-hour bus ride away, and we decide that the only way for me to find de time was to miss our next 'pointment and not miss my job at de farm. I decide not to call Amara to tell her and just show up real nice. I went to de local bakery and got her favorite lime cake, and I brought Mirlande's bike and her big sister Lovelie's favorite doll, which she done left behind they leave so fast. De bus driver must have thought I was on my way to a real good birtday party.

On de bus, it done felt like every family in de country was out there on de roadside. I was wonderin' if it were a warnin', like showin' me what I don't got because of all de things I done wrong. I thought, God done show me dose families are what you gone and lost because you done kill dat Buzzard. But den I thought, maybe it's God tellin' me there's good news ahead. I was getting' real confused and not feelin' so good. So I decided to leave God out of it. I tell myself dis was like a parade, and all dose families done come out and cheer me on. Den I fell asleep.

When I done get to town and find my way to deir house, Amara trew her arms around me, and my girls came runnin' and nearly done knocked me over de way kids do. Turns out Amara told dem de war was ragin' again and dat's why dey left. De girls dink I'm a hero back there protectin' their bike and doll. Amara's parents, dey okay to me, too. She hug, he shake my hand. We eat lunch togeta like dey knew I be comin'.

After, I talk wit Amara wit her daddy at her side and say it all 'gain what I done say on de phone. Her dad said she already done told 'em what I told her I on de phone and dat Rose don't sound like no healer. America don't got healers and whatever dis CBT ting is dat she knows and does to me, it ain't no healin'. I tell 'em it's not done to you, it's done wit you, but dat don't make 'em feel better. Den I asked dem what does it matter about Rose anyway—all dat matter is us, Amara and me?

Amara said it matter 'cause I not de same man she married. De war done changed me. She said, "You run with da Bustards and now you float around like a fish—your eyes open, but you be sleepin'."

Then I don't know why, but I just talked on and on: "Amara, I ain't been a sleepin' fish. I been a duck floatin' around real quiet but under de surface paddlin' away real hard. Before my mind can't stop—it goes and goes. Dat's why I done turned to de palm wine. It quiet dings. Now, de CBT, it quiet dings. It teach me how to dink de dings dat count and not dat don't count...." I paused and den I just went and said it: "Amara, I done killed a Buzzard! They made me do it! Dat's what I can't get off de mind!"

We didn't talk much about dings after dat and definitely not dat. Just light chitchat, and I spent de day playing wit de girls. I slept over and left de next day. But ever since we been talkin' on de phone.

I do believe we be back togetha sometime soon, me and my family. My derapy taught me I am not as wortless, as helpless, as unlovable as I gotten to believin'. Honest, I never really before been dinkin' about these things one way or de other—I just dink what I dink. But now I done seen what I dink and it don't control me no more. Dat give me energy and give me belief in who I am and it is dat belief what let me go visit Amara and de girls and start dings back down the right road for my family.

Talkin' to Amara, I dink she knew my secret all along and pretended to herself. I never knew you could hide tings from yourself, but I done learned from Rose you sure can. Sometimes that can be good, but mostly it be bad. And den you suffer from de unseen.

Epilogue

Summer's emerging from under the cover of the night as I walk, bringing the early morning to that moment when your outlook decides whether it's still cool or already hot. There's a sense of things to come in the absence of the urban crowds, which are massing somewhere out of sight. Parking meters far outnumber my fellow pedestrians, and a few joggers slalom around them as they quietly zip to-and-fro. A milk delivery truck suddenly rumbles by without consideration for the potholes or the serenity. And as I get to the hospital entrance, a faded gentleman sitting up against the building ignores the unspoken rule of silence and blurts "Got money?!" as he makes a subtle play at gatekeeping.

Patients already cram the clinic's still waiting room like students who rush to their seats before the teacher arrives. Barely able to wait for this party to start, the clinic managers wave me behind the reception desk into the office area. There's a lot of energy back here as the clinic hovers and shivers on the edge of the first appointments of the day. Start bringing the patients in!

I wish I could allow you to think I transformed Dr. Robinson's primary care clinic, but I am back home in America. Like the larger medical-student-driven primary care clinic within which it is situated, this is a mental health clinic staffed and run by medical students who are supervised with the lightest touch possible by a few faculty members at our medical school and a number of senior psychiatry residents who are selected to participate in our global mental health program. The residents' involvement ensures that their interest in improving access to mental health care is truly global and not just international, since neglected mental health needs do not just lie at the end of a valiant international quest but right outside the doors of our own temple of modern medicine. The mental health gap in our community yawns not so wide as to be mistaken for Mary's, but for each of our needlessly suffering community members, it may as well.

Remember what I said to Dr. Toussaint at the Ministry of Health about "making existing human resources more comfortable working with people with mental health problems and more knowledgeable and skilled in treating those problems"? Rose is the one-person embodiment of that aspiration, while this is an entire clinic founded on it. Student volunteers who are not yet doctors manage the clinic and provide medical and mental health care for an otherwise underserved, underinsured, and marginalized inner-city community. We only expect the students to treat patients with anxiety or depression, for which we even have CBT-trained student psychotherapists, and not those with what are usually more severe problems like manic depression or schizophrenia.

I am here to take my turn at supervising the student clinicians in the mental health clinic, and as it's my first time back since my trip to Doc Mary and company, I am operating in a compare-and-contrast frame of mind. As I duck my head into one consultation room after the other to lay eyes on things, I am reminded how similar our largely immigrant patients are to those who filled Dr. Robinson's clinic. Unemployment, food insecurity, homelessness, domestic violence, and long lists of medical problems are inevitable parts of the storylines of each and every patient and their families. They're not emerging from a war, but the guns and drugs on the street make it feel like they're in the middle of one. These parallels are a favorite teaching point of mine, but this trip placed me back in the role of student on the matter, part of my continuing re-education.

Our student-run, faculty-facilitated clinic relies on volunteer supervisors and student clinicians. It runs so well I call it a perpetual motion machine. One of my students even gave me a radiometer, the device once thought to be driven by perpetual motion but whose shaft and black and white vanes rotate under a glass bulb from the heat generated on the black panels by sunlight. Everybody gets something. The increasing number of medical students who select this as an extracurricular activity get an early entry to what they all came to medical school for—treating patients of their own. Public health and other allied health professional students who serve as clinical coordinators get immersed in a real-life public health experiment. Supervisors, most of whom are those senior residents or psychiatrists in training unlike me, get a head start on serving as supervising physicians. And patients get free mental health care on top of the free medical care they originally came for.

But we do require funding to pay for medications, which make up more than half of our clinic's overall budget, and we only serve about 75 patients/year, less than half of the overflowing inpatient census at what was Doc Mary's psychiatric hospital alone. And tens of thousands of dollars go toward paying the tuition of each of our student clinicians and the salaries of each of our resident supervisors so that they all have the extracurricular latitude to volunteer in our clinic. So, we're not quite a perpetual motion machine nor necessarily a translatable model for how to operate a country's public mental health system. But I think we do demonstrate the catalytic potential of believing, as I do, that access to mental health care is a right for everyone, everywhere.

The scarcity of mental health resources available to Mary and the Ministry of Health pales in comparison to what we have here at our medical school and here in the United States. I do not need to travel to such far-flung places in order to acknowledge this—after all, it is the very basis for going there in the first place. Like any other humanitarian lens through which America can and should look at the world around it, when it comes to mental health care we have more and should share, if not what we have then at least what we know. Mental health is not a luxury item of the developed world.

But Sam also drove home a point to me about scarcity and helped me reign in how much pity I take on those with less. His depression had nothing to do with how little he had. Neither his lifetime of bedless mattresses nor ill-fitting doors ever propelled him into depression—it was loneliness that got to him. First came the isolation he felt in his marriage for having committed murder as a Bustard conscript. Like so many who are traumatized, Sam felt alone with the memories of what he had done to the Buzzard, afraid or unwilling to share it and unburden himself off his guilt. Maybe he was afraid to traumatize Amara with this story; maybe he doubted she could understand; and maybe Sam felt he deserved to suffer for what he had done. But there's no doubting that Sam felt guilty for betraying Amara's trust after promising he would lay low among the Bustards and not participate in their violence, and he managed this guilt by holding his secret close.

Such so-called avoidant coping paved the way for shame, leaving Sam feeling not only that he had done something unforgivably wrong but that now there was something irrevocably wrong with him. Guilt and shame then nibbled away at him like a cancer of the soul, and he turned to alcohol as his chemotherapy. Maybe Amara would have reacted with no less fury had he told her of his crime early on than she did at his drinking and distancing and still fled to her mother's. But given that she fled anyway, Sam probably had nothing to lose in confessing his sin to her straight off and potentially averting the physical and even more profound isolation of her leaving with the girls. It was not his ramshackle home that eventually cast him into the abyss of depression but an empty one.

Support of all magnitudes proved to be a theme that ran through my trip. Sam was lacking for it until he met Londo, who proved humble enough to know that healing was an act and not a dogma and to assist Western healers like Mary and myself and the relentlessly helpful Molly. Berko and Ife literally wandered in the wilderness when their families shunned them out of fear and misunderstanding about Berko's mental illness. And Ife was the epitome of the supportive wife, honoring her marital vows when many would not and likely saving Berko from a tragic end. Even back here in the U.S., it was Molly's neighbor Virginia who appeared to be the linchpin of her bipolar mother's mental health plan in psychiatry-deficient rural America until Molly decided her mother needed her more than the world did.

It's hard to say whether Amara's understanding would have forestalled Sam's need for the likes of Rose, but it may have at least averted his descent into dual problems with alcoholism and depression. Likewise Ife was necessary for Berko's mental well-being, but not enough without Leridone.

Good support always hastens recovery from trauma, grief, and life's array of other departures from the futures we seek. But that support is not always enough to tug someone like Sam or Berko all the way out of the ditch. Mental health care—when it's available, affordable, and acceptable—can grab hold of the line to put its considerable heft behind the rescue.

About the Author

Craig L. Katz is a clinical professor of psychiatry, medical education, and system design and global health at the Icahn School of Medicine at Mount Sinai in New York, U.S.A.

When Dr. Katz was a chief resident in psychiatry at Columbia University/NYS Psychiatric Institute in 1998, Swissair Flight 111 crashed without survivors off of Nova Scotia after departing JFK *en route* to Paris. A request from the mayor's office seeking mental health professionals to assist families converging on JFK from around the world found its way to Columbia, and he and three other fellow residents were given leave to go to JFK, where they and but one other psychiatrist were the only mental health professionals. The experience of helping the families and the airline staff was a profound one. But when Dr. Katz and his colleagues got together to debrief among themselves over dinner, they realized not only that they felt ill-equipped by their training to deal with such acute trauma and grief but that their involvement was serendipitous. Nor was it clear under whose auspices they were working at JFK or at the crash site, to which several of his colleagues flew with families.

After consulting with the American Red Cross, what is now called the NYC Department of Health and Mental Hygiene, and a range of experts in psychology and psychiatry, they decided to found Disaster Psychiatry Outreach (DPO), an organization devoted to training and organizing psychiatrists to assist disaster-affected communities. They were assisted in this by a pro bono law firm that lost an associate in the crash.

Dr. Katz was the founding president of DPO and led it for the next eleven years. When 9/11 struck, DPO was able to partner with the City of New York to provide several hundred volunteer psychiatrists to assist at Ground Zero and the Family Assistance Center, initially at the Lexington Avenue Armory and then at Pier 94 on Manhattan's west side. Dr. Katz foresaw a need to be available in the long term to meet the mental health needs of the thousands of rescue and recovery workers and volunteers from Ground Zero. In a partnership between DPO and Mount Sinai, Dr. Katz was able to raise millions of dollars of private and eventually, federal funds to found and direct the WTC Mental Health Worker/Volunteer Mental Health Screening and Treatment Program. Dr. Katz directed this program for four years and supervised its social workers for many years thereafter; it continues to this day through federal funding and is now known as the WTC Health Program (https://www.mountsinai.org/care/occupational-health/services-programs/wtc). DPO became part of Vibrant Emotional Health organization in 2019 and is led by two of Dr. Katz's former residents (https://www.vibrant.org/what-we-do/advocacy-policy-education/crisis-emotional-care/).

Dr. Katz's involvement with DPO and especially with the response to 9/11 has led to several other developments in trauma and disaster response. In 2016, he was recruited by Advanced Recovery Systems and the International Association of Firefighters to help establish a specialized treatment center for traumatized firefighters in Maryland, The IAFF Center for Behavioral Healthcare Care Treatment and Recovery (https://www.iaffrecoverycenter.com/). He remains the National Trauma Consultant for ARS. He has also been part of the leadership of the Mount Sinai Human Rights Program since 2018, helping conduct psychiatric evaluations of asylum seekers from around the world and teaching others how to do so. And when the COVID-19 pandemic struck NYC, Dr. Katz was recruited to help establish and serve as a special adviser to a center for the mental health and well-being of his fellow healthcare workers in the Mount Sinai Health System during the pandemic, known as the Center for Stress, Resilience, and Personal Growth (https://icahn.mssm.edu/research/center-stress-resilience-personal-growth). Dr. Katz was awarded the American Psychiatric Association's Bruno Lima Award in Disaster Psychiatry in 2002 and the Medical Society of the State of New York's 2022 David B. L. Meza, III, MD Award for Excellence in Emergency Preparedness and Disaster/Terrorism Response.

From the very start of the co-founding of DPO, Dr. Katz was most interested in international disaster response. He therefore presided over and participated in disaster mental health missions to post-earthquake El Salvador in 2001 and post-tsunami Sri Lanka in 2005. It was during this last mission, on a visit to a stricken school to address the mental health needs of their traumatized and mourning students, that a teacher stood up and thanked the mental health team for coming, then politely asked where they had been before, as Sri Lanka had to deal with overwhelming mental health needs and scarce resources before the natural disaster. Looking at how much effort and planning it took to plan the trip to Sri Lanka, a country Dr. Katz and colleagues never had a chance to know except through the lens of disaster, and having learned from his WTC experience how important it was to remain involved not just in the acute aftermath of a disaster but potentially for years to come, Dr. Katz underwent a paradigm shift. He no longer wanted to show up after a disaster to affected communities, where his help seemed like too little, too late, but instead wanted to try to help improve access to mental health care in underserved communities in "normal times" and pursue mental health development work. In the thankfully rare event of a disaster, these communities would therefore be mentally healthier and therefore also better able to weather the event.

Dr. Katz's realization coincided with the founding of the Global Health Center at Mount Sinai by colleagues in emergency medicine, internal medicine, and pediatrics who were interested in global health service and education. They welcomed and supported his desire to pursue development work in mental health, and Dr. Katz was able to found the Mount Sinai Program in Global Mental Health in 2007 (https://icahn.mssm.edu/education/medical/global-health-opportunities/global-mental-health). Its mission: *The Program in Global Mental Health (GMH) at the Icahn School of Medicine at Mount Sinai (ISMMS) enhances access to mental health care for people in East Harlem and around the world. Our program develops, trains, and educates ISMMS students, residents, and faculty to provide mental health services to those who need them most.*

The Program in Global Mental Health began its work in Belize and over the years has grown to work across the globe including in Saint Vincent and the Grenadines, Haiti, Liberia, post-3/11 Japan (a remnant of Dr. Katz's disaster work), Costa Rica, Cape Verde, India, the Dominican Republic, Kenya, and Grenada. The program continues to work in most of the countries to this day, albeit remotely during the COVID-19 pandemic, and Dr. Katz has himself traveled to many of these countries, often leading the initial "needs assessment" trips that launch these partnerships. The program is not just international but also global, as it works in its own backyard in East Harlem and in immigrant detention centers in the United States. There are not many global mental health programs in the U.S., and those that exist tend to be research-focused. The Mount Sinai program is especially unique in having service as its primary mission, thinking of itself as a "walk-in mental health clinic" for the world. Indeed, most of the countries it works in have come about via "word of mouth," with a colleague in one country recommending Dr. Katz and his program to another country. In 2015, Dr. Katz was awarded the Mount Sinai Auxiliary Board Award for Outstanding Service in the International Community.

Fifty psychiatry residents and dozens of medical and graduate students have thus far graduated from the Program in Global Mental Health.

Dr. Katz has authored or co-authored 90 journal articles and book chapters on disaster psychiatry, global mental health, and human rights and has co-edited several books including *Disaster Psychiatry: Readiness, Evaluation, and Treatment* (APA Press, 2011), which has been translated into Korean and Japanese and is about to be released as a second edition. He co-founded in 2013 and still co-directs a graduate course in global mental health for Mount Sinai health professions students and psychiatry residents. In 2015, Dr. Katz and his former resident-turned-program-co-director, Dr. Jan Schuetz Mueller, decided to put their unique experience in global mental health into a book and co-authored *A Practical Guide to Global Mental Health: Seeing the Unseen* (Routledge, 2015).

Despite the Program in Global Mental Health and its many partners around the world, the "mental health gap" that exists between the level of need and availability of services around the world remains vast. Dr. Katz believes a narrative non-fiction book bringing alive people's stories and his own experiences in global mental health will not only prove captivating but also instrumental in narrowing that gap in a way that scientific papers cannot.

A native of Long Island, New York, Dr. Katz attended Harvard College and went on to Columbia University, where he obtained his medical degree, completed his psychiatric residency training, and served as chief resident in psychiatry. He subsequently completed a fellowship in forensic psychiatry at NYU. Dr. Katz has a private practice in general and forensic psychiatry in Manhattan and is a former president of the New York County District Branch of the American Psychiatric Association as well as a Distinguished Life Fellow of the APA. Dr. Katz is married to Linda, a pediatrician and a child psychiatrist who is herself Chair of the Disaster Committee of the American Academy of Child and Adolescent Psychiatry and is the proud father of 21-year-old Maya (who traveled with him to Haiti and Japan and plans to study international relations) and 18-year-old Lev (who traveled to Japan).